HOMEMADE SOAPS RECIPES:

Natural Handmade Soap, Soapmaking book with Step by Step Guidance for Cold Process of Soap Making

(How to Make Hand Made Soap, Ingredients, Soapmaking Supplies, Design Ideas)

Olivia Garden

Copyright © [Olivia Garden]

All rights reserved. No part of this guide may be reproduced in any form without permission in writing from the publisher except in the case of brief quotations embodied in critical articles or reviews.

Legal & Disclaimer

The information contained in this book and its contents are not designed to replace or take the place of any form of medical or professional advice; and is not meant to replace the need for independent medical, financial, legal, or other professional advice or services, as may be required. The content and information in this book have been provided for educational and entertainment purposes only.

The content and information contained in this book have been compiled from sources deemed reliable, and it is accurate to the best of the Author's knowledge, information, and belief. However, the Author cannot guarantee its accuracy and validity and cannot be held liable for any errors and/or omissions. Further, changes are periodically made to this book as and when needed. Where appropriate and/or necessary, you must consult a professional (including but not limited to your doctor, attorney, financial advisor or such other professional advisor) before using any of the suggested remedies, techniques, or information in this book.

Upon using the contents and information contained in this book, you agree to hold harmless the Author from and against any damages, costs, and expenses, including any legal fees potentially resulting from the application of any of the information provided by this book. This disclaimer applies to any of the loss, damages or injury caused by the use and application, whether directly or indirectly, of any advice or information presented, whether for breach of contract, tort, negligence, personal injury, criminal intent, or under any other cause of action.

You agree to accept all risks of using the information presented in this book.

You agree that, by continuing to read this book, where appropriate and/or necessary, you shall consult a professional (including but not limited to your doctor, attorney, or financial advisor or such other advisor as needed) before using any of the suggested remedies, techniques, or information in this book.

CONTENTS

- **INTRODUCTION TO HOME MADE SOAPS AND SOAP MAKING** 1
- **WHY YOU SHOULD MAKE YOUR OWN SOAP?** 2
- **SOAP MAKING SAFETY GUIDELINES** 4
- **SOAP MAKING METHODS** 7
  - Melt and pour Method 7
  - The Rebatching Method 9
  - The Hot Process 10
  - The Cold Process 10
- **CHOOSING EQUIPMENT** 17
- **SOAP MAKING INGREDIENTS** 19
- **DECORATING YOUR SOAP** 21
- **RECIPES** 23
  - Quick and simple 4 oil soap recipe 24
  - Olive Oil Soap for Baby sensitive skin 25
  - Creamy and Luxurious soap Recipe 27
  - Lavender Heaven 29
  - Green Tea with Eucalyptus and Lemon Grass Nature's Blend 31
  - Coffee Soap Recipe 33
  - Healthy Classical Pine Tar soap 35
  - Pampering Shea and Cocoa Butter Recipe 37
  - Pumpkin Spice Soap 39
  - Goat Milk with coloured Glitter 41
  - Refreshing and Soothing Cucumber Blend 43
  - Coconut Milk Soap 45
  - Tea Tree and Charcoal Soap 47
  - Clover and Aloe 49
  - Coconut Oil Soap (Beginners recipe) 51
  - Lavender and Goat Milk Soap 52
  - Oat Meal Soap 54
  - Zesty Lemon Soap 56
  - Orange Zest Soap 58
  - Tea and Peppermint Soap 60
  - French Green Clay Soap 62
  - Vanilla Soap 64
  - Rose Water Petal Soap 66

Sea Mud and Cedar Wood Soap 68
Chai Vanilla Soap 70
Apple Cinnamon Winter Soap 72
Loofa Soap 74
Yogurt and Banana Flax Seed Soap 76
Lemon and Poppy Soap 78
Raspberry Soap 80

CONCLUSION..82

Introduction to Home Made Soaps and Soap Making

Many people are under the impression that they can't make their own soap at home. The truth is that you CAN make your own soap at home. It is a much more rewarding experience to do your own soap at home than to buy commercial soap. This book will shine light on the concept of "Do it yourself" soap and guide you on how to safely and elegantly experiment and create your own soap at home using very basic ingredients.

Making soap is about chemistry, using the right ingredients in the right proportions. What if you are not a chemist? Don't worry, this book is designed to be a beginners' guide, explaining in a simplified manner the chemistry of soap making, while providing recipes with instructions that you can easily follow along whilst leaving sufficient scope for you to get creative with the soap making process. With this book, you are in good hands, just like how your hands will be when you make your own natural soup.

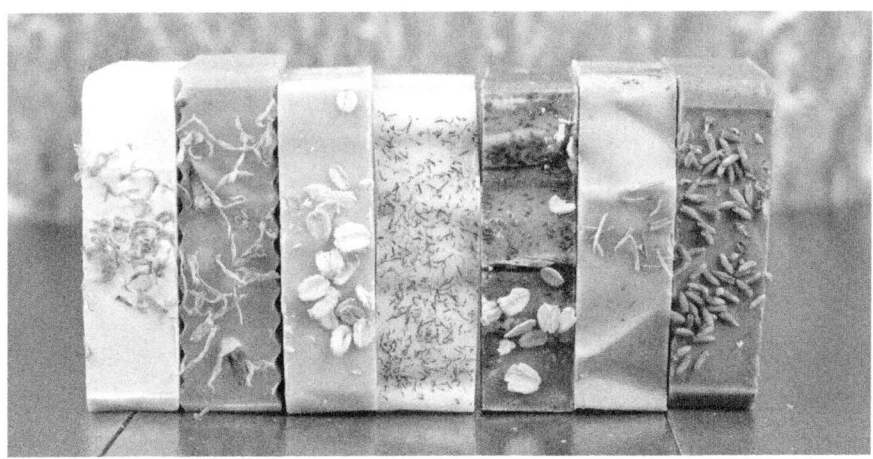

WHY YOU SHOULD MAKE YOUR OWN SOAP?

Soap sold commercially is most often made on a large scale with the most cost effective way possible. This includes using chemical detergents, hardening material and other chemicals that are very harmful to your skin. The chemicals in commercial soap often leave your hands dry as they focus on cleaning and forget about pampering your skin. When you make homemade soap, it is made with natural ingredients such as lye and natural oils. Moreover, you can also control what you add in there, for example, adding natural aromatherapy oils or compounds such as glycerin. Glycerin is a small amino acid that is very good for the softness of your skin. The process of soap making naturally produces glycerin. However, most commercial soaps don't have glycerin. That is because they extract it to make use of it for other skin loving and high-quality products such as moisturizing lotions. This leaves the soap hard and irritating to the skin, although it cleans well. But soap also needs to be skin loving and soft on the skin. With natural homemade soap, you can add glycerin or whatever skin friendly ingredient you want to add.

You may argue that homemade soap uses lye and you don't want lye on your skin. The wonder of chemistry is that during the process of saponification, the lye completely dissolves and reacts with the oils used to form soap, and no more lye remains if you have used the correct proportions.

One of the best advantages of making your own soap is that you can be sure of all the ingredients included. You are 100% in control. You can choose to use all-natural products, even the coloring can be used from natural and skin friendly alternatives.

Another beauty of making your own soap is that you are the master of the process. You can control how you want your soap to feel. Do you want to make it soft or hard? What scent do you want your soap to have? Do you want your soap to be frothy and lathery or have little lather? All this you can control by adjusting the proportions of lye and the type of oils you use. For example, using castor oil gives you different results than when using olive oil and so on and so forth. The possibilities are almost endless with homemade soap. Think of all the experimenting fun you can have!

Soap making can be a life changing activity. DIY soap is a fun and relaxing activity to do to release stress. Therefore, it is a great outlet to de-stress and try something new. It is also an outlet to feel different or discover a new hobby. It is a great opportunity to express and discover your creativity by experimenting with different proportions, ingredients and add ons. Moreover, you can always get creative with the shapes of the molds, colour combinations, petal additions and even the final packaging. It would also be perfect as a bonding arts and crafts activity. Your homemade soap will make you feel proud about your achievement and progress as you can see your bathroom shelves stacked with the magical work of your hands.

Soap making can also be your chance to increase your income as you can make handmade soap and sell it, making your own brand by using your own creative touch. Homemade soap has helped a lot of females take care of their families by selling the soap they make. Moreover, it is a creative and a wonderful sensual gift to give your friends, family or loved ones. There are tons of reasons to make your own soap, without further ado, let's get into HOW you can make your own soap. But before that, as always, safety first, so let us discuss some safety considerations while making soap at home.

SOAP MAKING SAFETY GUIDELINES

Safety is always first. Working with Lye and inducing a chemical reaction entails taking caution when attempting such procedures.

Research about your ingredients to understand what you are working with

Before you start, it is highly advised that you take your time to understand your ingredients. We will be explaining more about the ingredients in the coming chapters. For example, Lye is a substance to be treated with care. Spend some time getting to know about it for example, if you spill lye solution, don't attempt to neutralize it with vinegar. Instead, you need to rinse it with excess water. Whether it splashed in your eyes or mouth or on your skin, rinsing it with water is the only and best solution to avoid skin or eye injury. If it spills on your clothes, remove the affected clothes immediately.

Follow your Recipe

Chemical reactions need to occur in a certain way. It is all about proportions. Too much or too little of something can result in an undesirable effect. In soap making, all recipe ingredients are mentioned by weight, often ounces as you use traces of each ingredient. Therefore, it would be great if have your recipe printed-out so you can make sure of it, instead of fumbling with the phone or tablet while working with your ingredients, especially lye, you might risk spilling something. It may take you a couple of times to memorize the recipe by heart and then it would be much easier.

The second thing you need to follow your recipes precisely is a sensitive scale. Get a good quality kitchen scale or a digital scale. Make sure you test it out first with other known weights, such as a coin of known weight to confirm your balance's accuracy. Once tested, you need to weigh out all your ingredients as per your recipe. It is not advised to alter to change anything in the beginning. Some recipes mention percentages rather than weights which you can use to modify recipes according to your desired quantity but in the beginning, it is best to test with a prewritten recipe.

Take Care of Your Eyes

Your eyes should be one of your number one safety priorities. A lot of things could go wrong and enter your eye during soap making, however, you can overcome this problem by wearing safety lab goggles. Lye or raw soap or dye powder all could find their way into your eyes, but not if you had safety goggles on. You should never skip this step. You also need close-by access to water to wash it just in case. If you want maximum visibility, consider anti-fog goggles.

Take Care of your skin

Just like your eyes, the same is true for your skin. Lye or raw soap can be highly irritant to your skin if you were not wearing protective gloves. You can use latex gloves or rubber gloves. Dishwashing gloves are also fine but they can be bulky to work with. You could also protect your skin by wearing an apron or long sleeved top so that you don't have your skin exposed.

Ventilate your Room

It is not advisable to work with a chemical reaction and the raw soap smell with closed windows. Keep the windows opened in the room that you are in to breathe fresh air.

Be Prepared for Spills

Even if you wear protective gear, anything could happen. That is why it is always important to have a plan B. Buy a granular absorbent or a universal absorbent spill kit and have this nearby.

The spill could be oil, your soap, lye, etc. Always keep a water supply nearby.

Make Sure You Have Printed the Right Recipe Without Any Errors

Sometimes people can write anything on the Internet without having the appropriate knowledge of the percentages and calculations. Make sure you get recipes from trusted sources. You can use the recipes in this book.

Prepare All Your Ingredients before Hand

When you start, there isn't then time to go around your kitchen gathering or weighing the rest of your ingredients. Keep everything ready and within hands reach before you start.

Work with a Clear Space

Clutter is always a huge obstacle in any process. With lots of clutter, the chances of error increase. Always keep a clear working space.

Record Your Results and Learn from Your Mistakes

It is important to record the results of your batches so that you can figure out what went wrong and avoid it in the future.

- Keep Pets and Children Away
- Label the Utensils You Used For Lye
- Be cautious but don't let that inhibit your creativity to decrease your fun

Soap Making Methods

There are many methods to make soap, some are quite easy while others are an art; a complex art, but not impossible.

Melt and pour Method

This is one of the easiest soap making processes and saves quite a lot of time. In this process, you can use a premade soap base that has undergone the saponification process rather than spend time mixing fats with an alkali such as lye, which can be time consuming as it requires more preparation time. A readymade soap base contains glycerin and fatty acids as well as other natural ingredients.

The melt and pour method is the perfect choice if you are a beginner, still exploring the arena and would like to play it safe. All you have to do is purchase pre-made solid soap base instead of making it from scratch and you are ready to use the soap once it hardens, no unnecessary waiting for a cure time to pass such as with cold process.

How this method works:

Head to a nearby arts and crafts store and look for a premade soap base. One of the best options to purchase are the clear glycerin or white premade soap bases. Don't use a bar of soap for this as it is not the same thing and will give you trouble while melting.

The next step would be to melt your solid premade soap base. To speed up this process, use a sharpened knife to cut the bar into small 1-inch chunks. Don't worry about exact measurements here. The goal is to have smaller pieces rather than one large chunk as smaller pieces will melt faster.

In a microwave, add your cut chunks in a microwave friendly dish and heat for 30 seconds. Take out the dish and stir your melted contents then reheat again for another 30 seconds then take out to stir again. Repeat this cycle of 30 seconds heat then stir until you feel the consistency of your melted soap base as completely liquidy with no lumps or hard chunks in between. That is when your entire soap base has melted. Don't overheat it beyond that point.

Some people don't own a microwave in their house, it is possible to replace it with a saucepan filled with water to create a water bath. Heat the water and then put a glass bowl and let it float in the hot water. Put your soap base chunks in the glass bowl and watch it melt through the heat that transfers from the hot water to the glass bowl and consequently to the soap base chunks that melt eloquently. Don't forget to stir. Remove the bowl from the sauce pan when your soap base has completely melted and doesn't have any lumps.

Let your soap melt to cool down to around 50 degree Celsius. Do not add your essential oils or dye while the melt is still hot. Likewise, don't let it cool to the point of hardening. Add 2-3 drops of your desired dye depending on the colour intensity you desire. If you are using a powdered dye, dissolve 2-3 teaspoons of your powdered dye in some liquid glycerin as you can't add the power directly to your melt or else the colour will not get distributed evenly. It is always wonderful to add a pleasant scent to your soap. For 1 pound of soap, you can add 1 tablespoon of fragrance oil or half a tablespoon of essential oil. Make sure you use the ones labelled for soap making and not candle oils, to ensure they are friendly and soft on your skin.

Stir all your added dye and fragrance drops before the last step. The last step would be to pour your coloured and fragranced melt into a mold of your choice then let it cool naturally for 12-24 hours. When your soap has completely solidified, take it out of the mold and it would be ready for use immediately. However, make sure the edges have dried completely.

The Rebatching Method

A similar quick and easy method is the rebatching method. As the name suggests, it is often used to rebatch (make use of the soap you did) if there were any mistakes or if you didn't like the shape of the mold or messed it up during the design process. You can also use this method if you want to get a taste of the soap making DIY experience without buying additional equipment. In that cause, you can use pre existing soap. However, readymade soap never melts easily, that is why, although you will heat it as we described in the melt and pour method, you will add few table spoons of water, glycerin, etc to soften up the mix, then with heat resistant gloves, you will add your soap melt in a Ziploc bag and knead it so make it into a mushy texture.

Similar to the melt and pour process, you can add the dye and fragrance to your mix in the rebatching method and then let it solidify. This will take 5-7 days however as you wait for all the water to evaporate. Don't get impatient and use the freezer. Rebatched soap does not have the most aesthetic look or feel, but it is a suitable solution to ruined soap or if you want to add your own colour and fragrance to existing soap. Moreover, this method bypasses the drawback of adding stuff that get ruined by lye such as lavender buds that turn brown with lye. You can also use colours that are sensitive to the pH of lye that you can't use in the cold process. Similar is the case with being able to use light fragrances with the rebatching method which get masked when used in the cold process.

The benefits of both rebatching and melt and pour methods is that you don't have to deal with lye, which is feared by many people as it is a strong alkali. Moreover, you don't even need a lot of ingredients to start with or complex calculations and you can immediately get to enjoying the soap once it solidifies. However, on the other hand, you have very little control over the raw ingredients used as you are starting with something that someone else made, you don't control everything from scratch as with the cold method. If you would like to be the master of the experiment and totally in control of what goes in your soap, then the cold process is the best process for you.

THE HOT PROCESS

This process is like the cold process but involves using heat pots and "cooking" the soap rather than doing it cold.

THE COLD PROCESS

Keep in mind that in soap making, the cold process is the dragon level of all levels. The game play becomes a little bit more complex, but don't worry we have got your back and we are here to guide you through it step by step. The reward here is that there are unlimited possibilities to how you can make your final product in terms of colours, shapes and natural additions. Moreover, you can 100% guarantee that your soap is home made from scratch.

Let us start with the basic ingredients you will need for making soap using the cold process:

Lye flakes and clean distilled water

A source of fat, whether animal fat or vegetable oil

A natural soap dye of your choice, whether liquid or powder (optional but preferred)

Soap pot along with other equipments which we will discuss in more details shortly

Fragrance or an essential oil of your choice (optional but preferred)

A mold of your desired shape

A clean environment to work in and a cool dry place to let the soap cure in

For aesthetics petals or exfoliates (optional)

A handy recipe to follow (we will provide you with one)

How It Works:

The essence of the cold soap making process is preparing lye and a source of fat and mixing it together

1- Making the Lye solution

The first step is to prepare the lye solution. For exact amounts, you will have to refer to your chosen recipe.

Using your kitchen scale or digital scale, place the glass pitcher and set the scale to zero. Next you would be adding distilled water as per indicated in your recipe. Some recipes indicate weight; therefore you will place the pitcher on the scale. Other recipes indicate volume; therefore you can use your measuring cup.

Next it is time to measure up the lye. Do so using your mason jar with a tight secure lid. Lye is an alkali and is dangerous to your skin. That is why you need to handle it using gloves and while wearing your safety goggles. If any lye flakes cling to your glove, remove them immediately. Place the Mason jar and its lid on the scale and set it to zero. Add in the lye flakes until the scale indicates the weight indicated in your chosen recipe. You can replace the Mason jar with a plastic pitcher. However, don't use this pitcher for anything else except handling lye during your soap making process.

After your weights are set as per indicated in your recipe, time to mix them up. But be careful about this step. Take care to add the lye to the water bit by bit and not pour the water to the lye. Gently start adding your lye flakes to the pitcher containing water. Add it bit by bit from a close but safe distance to avoid splashes. To dissolve the lye appropriately, stir the mixture gently and slowly, again without splashing. As the two react, you will start to hear fizzing sounds or feel heat which is normal. Don't let the solution touch your skin directly. Keep your goggles and gloves on. Wash the item you used to stir with immediately after stirring. Don't forget to cover your pitcher containing your newly mixed lye water and let it settle for some time. Make sure it is tied securely and placed in a safe place away from pets or children. Caution should always be in mind around lye or lye water.

2- Preparing the oils

Get your handy scale again because we will weigh out your chosen oil as per the recipe, using the same method of adding the soap pot or a glass pitcher on the scale and setting it to zero. It is preferred to use the soap pot to weigh solid oils such as cocoa butter while using the glass pitcher for liquid oil such as olive oil. Slowly add the oil to your container till the scale hits the desired weight.

Examples of solid fat sources: Cocoa butter, coconut or palm

Examples of liquid fat sources: Castor oil, canola oil, olive oil, sunflower oil

If you are using a solid oil, melt it first using a sauce pan. This will shorten the step for you as you need to heat your chosen oil anyway. The oil needs to heat gradually, so apply medium heat and stir gently. You need to watch the temperature of your oil using the thermometer and turn off the heat when it reaches about 110 F. However, you can't add it just yet to the lye water mixture. The oils temperature needs to drop to 100 F before it can be mixed with the lye water. If you are using solid oil, make sure all the solid oil has come to a melt. If your recipe indicates a mixture of solid and liquid oils, add the liquid oils after all the solid fats melts. However, monitor your temperature again as this will lower the temperature of the overall oil mixture. Remember, you need it to be around 100 F when you mix it with the lye water.

3- Add the Lye water to the Oil base

Once you mix these two, the saponification reaction will be instant, and the mixture will turn cloudy, indicating a chemical reaction where the lye and oil react in the presence of heat to make soap. The lye is no longer chemically lye that is why handmade soap is safe on the skin, it no longer contains lye as it all transformed to soap when it mixed with the hot oil. Because from here on the process will happen quickly, you need to have your desired additions on standby, for example your fragrance bottles, essential oils, dye, spatulas, etc.

Gently add the lye mixture to the hot oil in the soap pot. You will notice a colour change and that the mixture will start to be cloudy. Stir gently, preferably with a stick blender, although, keep it turned off at this point. After you have poured in all your lye water mixture, keep the glass pitcher that contained it in a safe spot for the time being until you safely clean it later. Right now, you need to stay with your new mixture.

If you are using a stick blender, turn it on now and let it mix the mixture in short bursts of a few seconds and repeat until you feel that both your lye water and oil have completely mixed until you reach trace. Trace is reached when the mixture has emulsified, meaning, when the mixture is left later, it will keep getting thicker and thicker with time as part of the process.

How to Know If You Have Reached Trace Point?

The stick blender has severely quickened the process of saponification and reaching trace takes seconds compared to hours using regular stirring. If your mixture still has glistening oily liquidly floating between strokes, then all the oil has not mixed completely with your lye water yet. You will reach trace when the creamy consistency starts to slightly thicken and has a uniform consistency instead of having both thick and oily consistencies.

Why Is It Important to Reach Trace Point?

For many reasons, chief among them is that since tracing point is the point where all the mixture has emulsified and became soap particles instead of oil and lye, that means pouring the mixture before achieving trace results in having incomplete soap. This will lead to deformed soap or incompletely formed soap. Moreover, you will still have lye particles in your soap which will be very harmful to your skin. Therefore, you need to keep stirring until you have a think cake-like batter consistency with no glistening oil streaks. This mixture will also be easy to pour into a mold and will be of uniform consistency, you won't find oil dripping from the batter

It is safe to add your dye and fragrance in the light trace step before the thick medium trace step begins. Medium trace has a thicker consistency than light trace, resembling that of a pudding consistency. You can test for it by trickling some of the batter from the blender and it will form visible soap streaks on the mixture's surface the way chocolate streaks on a cake. This is the most suitable time to add your natural hard additives such as leaves, exfoliate, petals, etc.

The final trace consistency is that which resembles a thick pudding batter. That is the trace consistency that will conform to its shape when poured into a mold and that is what you want. To reach this trace stage, you need to keep stirring with the stick blender. If you want to create soap frosting, you will need to extremely thicken your trace to get soap consistency for frosting or decorative purposes.

Keep in mind a very important false trace sign. When you use a solid trace, if it has not been thoroughly melted and heating, it can easily cool during the mixing process and give the false sensation of hardening mixture while in fact it is not hardening due to saponification but it is due to hardening of the solid fat. For that reason, make sure to adequately heat it.

Factors That Can Affect Trace Consistency

There is no doubt that using a stick will make you reach a medium and thick consistency trace faster than stirring by hand. If you would like to give your dye and fragrance some time to mix, consider stirring by hand using a spatula when you reach thin trace consistency.

Some fragrances and additives such as clay speed up the trace process and make your mixture thicken fast. Be mindful about such additions and the timing and method of stirring. It is preferred to switch to manual stirring after adding a fragrance.

4- Adding your personal touch to the batter

After reaching your desired state, and before it is too thick, you can now add your chosen fragrance, essential oils and additives such as herbs, petals or natural exfoliants. Then gently stir and make sure your additions are thoroughly mixed within the batter. We will discuss some examples of exfoliants and essential oils.

Coloring your Soap

One of the most beautiful aspects of making your own soap is that you can choose the colour of your soap. You can have your colour as one solid colour for the entire bar or you can get creative with colour streaks. If you want to have a simply coloured bar of soap, add your desired colour dye, few drops or ½ a tea spoon into the batter. Make sure it is soap dye and not candle dye. You can add more dye to increase the colour intensity of the soap but don't overdo it. Stir well to evenly distribute the colour.

If you want to try creative methods such as the streak method, get about half a cup or a cup of your soap separately in your measuring cup and add the dye to it and mix thoroughly. Put the rest of your soap batter in your desired mold and gently pour your coloured mixture to the corner of the mold. Using a wooden or rubber spatula, start pulling coloured streaks from the coloured corner to design the soap batter that is lying in the mold away from the corner. You can swirl around the colour to create your desired pattered but don't overdo it so that you don't blend the colour with the entire mixture. You can use a Lazy Susan to try swirling techniques. The beauty of this step is that you can get very creative with colour designs and patterns or even colour combinations of your choice.

Pour your Mixture into a mold

By now, your mixture is ready to be poured into your desired mold. As you would evenly pour a cake mix into a mold, do so with your soap batter. A handy rubber spatula will aid you to scrape off the rest of the soap batter in your soap pot and into the mold. Finally, shake the mold gently to evenly distribute the soap batter in your mold to get a uniform bar. To get a soap bar with a smooth surface, you need to smooth out the surface of the mixture and even it out with the back of a spoon or with a rubber spatula.

Sometimes air bubbles would accumulate in your mixture during the pouring step. You will need to get rid of those. Gently tap your mold against the kitchen top to release any bubbles. Finally, leave your soap to cure in a warm and a safe place.

Now it is time to leave your mold for about 24 hours to harden. After this period of time, it would be ready to take it out of the mold and slice it into acceptable size bars. It is best to keep those bars to cure for 4 weeks before using it although it is safe to use right away. Meanwhile, don't forget to wash all the equipment you used very well with hot water and soap while still wearing your gloves and goggles.

Choosing Equipment

Goggles and Rubber gloves

Safety is always first. You cannot skip these essential items of equipment at all. Make sure you wear protective gloves for your hands and protective eye goggles for eye protection to protect against the irritant lye solution and during mixing soap.

Spatulas and spoons for stirring

You will need rubber ones for scraping off the last bits of mix from the soap pot. You will also need wooden ones for stirring. Plastic could also work but make sure it is heat resistant to resist the heat emitted when the saponification reaction takes place.

A digital scale or a kitchen scale for measuring and measuring cups

Accurate measurement of ingredients is the key to nailing the soap recipe successfully. You need a sensitive scale to accurately measure the weight of lye, distilled water, oils and even dye powder.

Soap Pot

You can use stainless steel or plastic large pots. It is better to have large pots so that you mix everything at once, instead of making smaller batches. This is the pot you will use for mixing your soap.

Thermometer

You need to be able to quickly and accurately measure the temperature of oils and the lye water

Mold

The soap making process is not complete without pouring your mixture into a mold. You can purchase a specific soap mold or you can use any house old item that fits the purpose such as an old yoghurt containers or plastic containers.

Stick Blender

To start the saponification process and reach the trace, you need a hand blender that will speed up the saponification process. You can stir by hand but that would take hours.

Measuring Cups

You will need various containers for measuring up your ingredients before weighing them or for measuring your dye and fragrance.

Glass pitcher

This is for mixing lye; it is preferred to label it "Hazardous" to indicate caution and to ensure people stay away from it. You may need another one to weigh in and heat your oil in.

Additional

You may need professional soap cutters to cut out the bars. You may also need stamps for decorative purposes or for professional labeling.

Soap Making Ingredients

Lye

It is sodium hydroxide, an alkali substance used in oven cleaners etc. It is caustic and highly irritant, but it is critical to the saponification process. Lye can result from the white ashes of extremely burnt wood at very high temperatures. It is used in drain cleaners. Don't buy drain cleaners to use for the soap making process. Buy the raw lye. Make sure you buy 100% lye. To ensure a pure product, buy it directly from the manufacturer.

Oils

The type of oil affects the hardness and lather of the soap. The combination of oils you chose for the soap can be optimized to achieve the hardness or softness you want.

Coconut Oil- Hard, lots of lather, makes the soap drying. Add more fat to soften the soap, although it gives good consistency.

Palm Oil- Hard, makes a long-lasting bar. Mild lather. Great alternative to animal fat.

Olive oil- Soft, low cleansing effects, and offers a slippery lather. Castile soap is 100% olive oil. It is suitable for sensitive skin. Takes a longer time to cure and harden. It is better to use extra virgin oil.

Lard- Hard, has a creamy lather. 100% lard can be a great laundry soap.

Cocoa butter- brittle and long-lasting bar. Creamy lather.

Shea Butter- Hard, medium creamy lather, long-lasting bar.

Castor oil- Improves the lather by improving soap solubility.

Other options- Avocado oil, almond oil, palm kernel oil.

Fragrances and Essential Oils

Fragrance oil is a mixture of natural and synthetic, carefully blended after lots of trials to provide an alluring and captivating scent. Many of them are thinned and diluted to have the perfume/scent quality. There are safe soap fragrance oils that are safe to your skin but make sure it is designed for soap to ensure its safety.

Essential oils are natural and made from plants by capturing the essence of the plant. The oil can be taken from various parts of the plant, depending on the plant. It can be seeds or leaves. Fragrances and essential oils are a wonderful addition to your product. Experiment with different oils. Some recipes guide you which oils to use. You can use either or a mix of both.

Herbs, Roots, Flowers, Petals, Fruits

Some recipes make use of herbs such as tea, lavender or even coffee beans. Keep your mind open to new variations. You can dice up fruit such as pumpkins or grate cucumber peel to add a beautiful touch.

Colorants

It is a wonderful addition to add color to your soap. Lavender smelling soap could be coloured purple to compliment the mental image. Some recipes offer natural colouring like cucumber infused recipes.

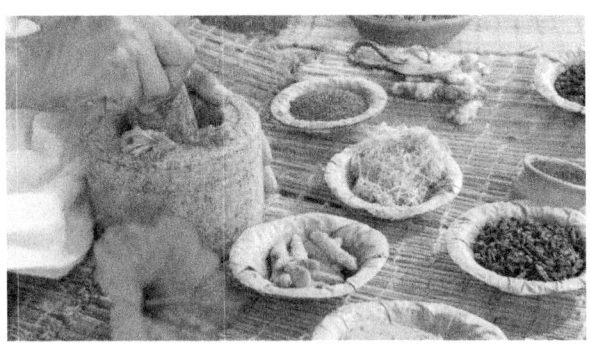

Decorating your Soap

You can get very creative with your soap, starting with picking the shape of the mold or creating your own mold. Another great method would be to swirl the soap or use certain dividers in a way that creates new designs. The malleability of soap allows you to make it into any shape you desire easily. You can even cut the soap into small heart shaped pieces and put them in a jar with a cute note or shape it as cookies or anything you literally want.

Coloring is another great thing to get creative with when designing. You can create master pieces and colour combinations. It is a great idea to have inspiration on how to design your soap.

You can also use the edge of the spoon to engrave patterns in the soap, insert petals, rhinestones, glitter, herbs, secret message inside. Literally anything you want. Certain petals can add a luxurious touch to your soap. It is really up to your creativity. You can also buy a stamp that makes cute shapes on the surface of the soap or engraves your trademark.

The packaging of the soap itself is an important factor in how professional and appealing your soap looks. Make sure the soap edges are cut neatly and smoothly as well as evenly. Invest in some creative and cute packing, make it personal and make it lovely.

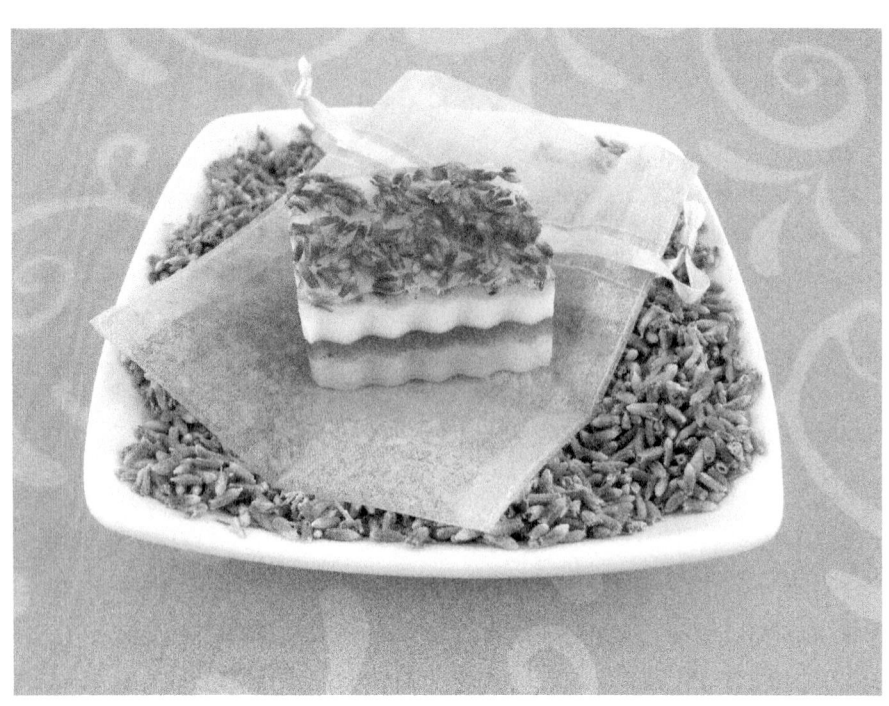

RECIPES

Refer to details of the soap making process in the cold process section. However, here are the steps again for simplicity.

Weigh your ingredients using the scale

Add the lye to the pitcher containing water (not the other way around) and stir to make a lye solution

Heat the oils to 110 F

Add the lye solution to the oil when they are at 100 F and stir

Using a stick blender, mix the mixture in short bursts until you achieve trace

Add your fragrance or essential oils

Pour your soap mixture into your chosen mold and let it harden for 12-24 hours to solidify

You can use the soap immediately, but it is better to let it cure for 3-4 weeks

Don't forget to adequately wash the equipment and utensils used

Use this method for all the following recipes.

Prep time for all recipes is appx. 60-120 minutes

QUICK AND SIMPLE 4 OIL SOAP RECIPE

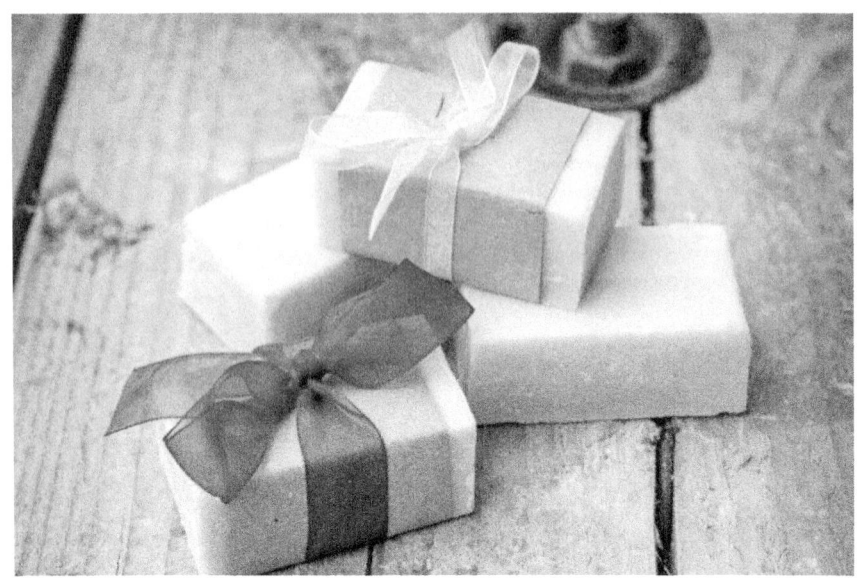

The oils

7.5 ounces olive oil

6.5 ounces palm oil

1.3 ounces castor oil

6.5 ounces coconut oil

The Lye Mixture

3.1 ounces lye

8 ounces water

Personal Additions

1 ounces of your favorite fragrance oil or any essential oil blend

Petals or exfoliants if desired

Olive Oil Soap for Baby sensitive skin

The high olive oil concentration makes this recipe soft and mild on your baby's skin. It is nourishing as well. However, the soap may need longer time to cure as the olive oil will make the soap take its time to harden but it will be worth it in the end as it will appeal to your baby's soft and sensitive skin.

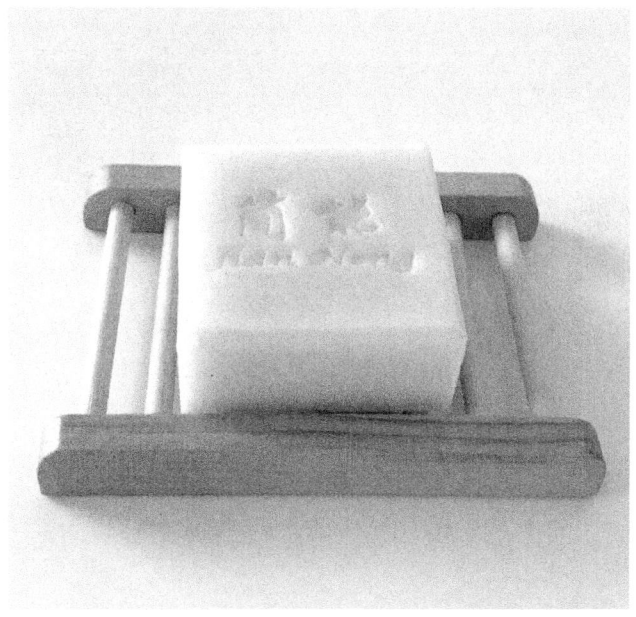

This recipe can make 12 bars, 3.6 pounds each

The Oils

2.1 ounces 5% Castor oil

6.2 ounces 15% coconut oil

28.7 ounces regular or infused 70% Olive oil

4.1 ounces 10% Shea Butter

For the Lye solution

5.48 ounces Lye

10.6 ounces water

2 teaspoons of Sugar added to the lye solution

1.5 teaspoons of Salt added to the lye solution

Additions

Optional, depending on how sensitive your baby's skin is

1.8 ounces Fragrance or essential oil

Creamy and Luxurious soap Recipe

Any soap recipe that includes milk is known to be super moisturizing and gives your soap a luxurious creamy touch. You can replace the water in your lye solution with milk either entirely or use half water and half milk when dissolving the lye. You can also use powdered milk that you add during the trace step. Either ways, this is a wonderful recipe if you suffer from dry skin.

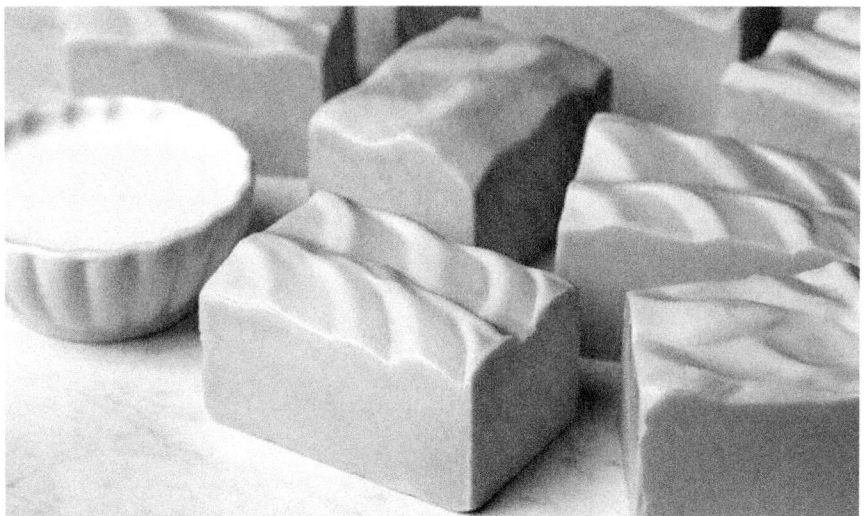

The oils

2.75 ounces 14% almond oil

1 ounce 5% castor oil

5.3 ounces 27% olive oil

5.3 ounces 27% palm oil

5.3 ounces 27% coconut oil

For the Lye solution

2.8 ounces of lye

5.9 ounces of water

Additional

1 ounce fragrance oil

Note: You can make half the 5.9 water and half of it milk. If you decide to use liquid milk, add the milk with the lye solution. If you decided to use heavy cream instead of milk, add it with the oils

LAVENDER HEAVEN

This heavenly recipe is admired by many due to its magical aroma. Follow the usual cold process soap making steps. Add the ingredients titled under "the magic touch" at trace. Let your wonder soap cure for 3-4 weeks. Add colorants if desired. The blend of patchouli along with the orange essence and lavender gives this recipe a distinctive touch

This recipe makes about 3 pounds of lavender infused soap

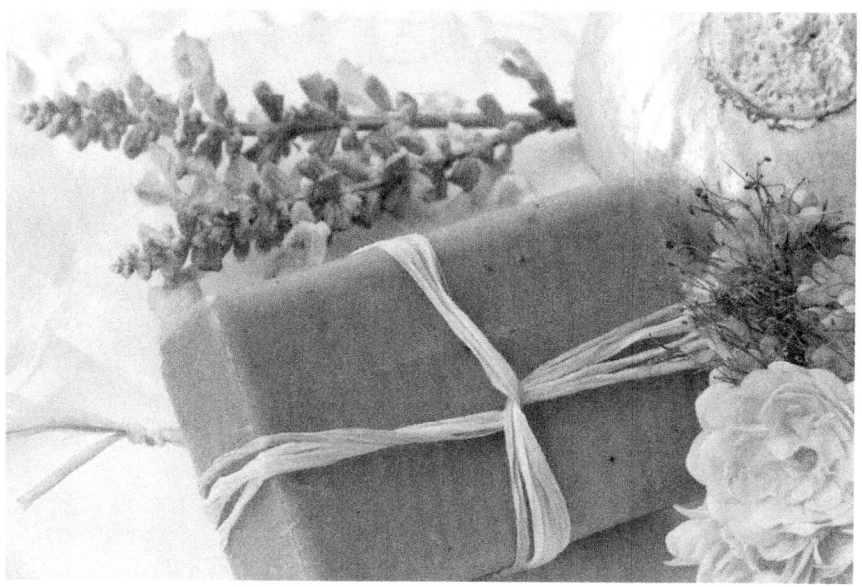

The oils

10.2 ounces of coconut oil

10.2 ounces of olive oil

3.4 ounces of sunflower oil

1.7 ounces of cocoa butter

1.7 ounces of castor oil

6.8 ounces of palm oil

For the Lye solution

4.9 ounces of lye

11.3 ounces of water

The magic touch

2 tbsp. of lightly ground lavender buds

0.8 ounces of lavender essential oil

0.5 ounces of orange essential oil

0.3 ounces of patchouli essential oil

GREEN TEA WITH EUCALYPTUS AND LEMON GRASS NATURE'S BLEND

What if I tell you that you can make use of the benefits of green tea in your soap so that your hands get some of its benefits too? Well, you can. This recipe allows you to include the magic of brewed green tea and green tea leaves in your soap. Follow the usual cold process soap making steps. Add the ingredients titled under "the magic touch" at trace. Let your wonder soap cure for 3-4 weeks. Add colorants if desired. A light green color would reflect and match with the aroma of the soap.

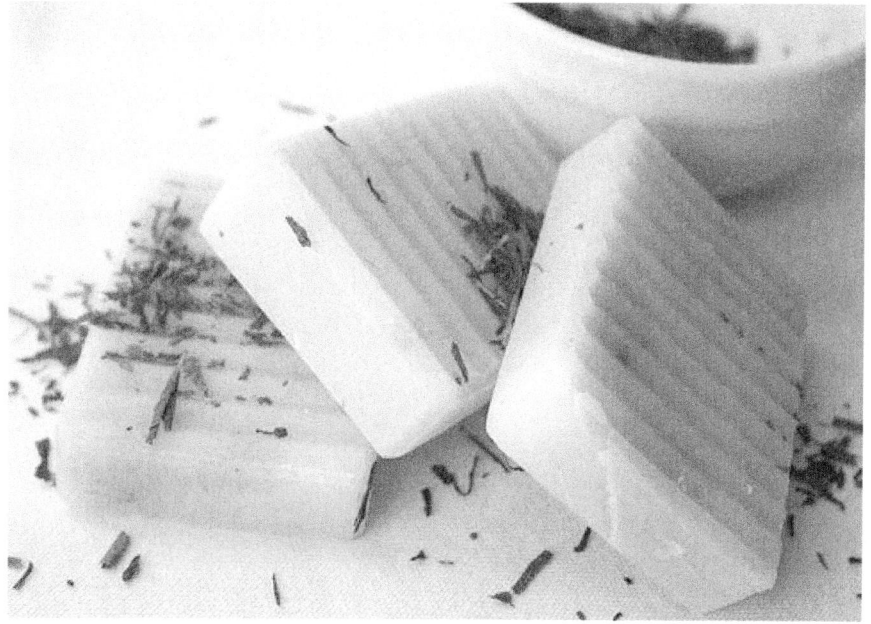

The oils

11 ounces of olive oil

5.2 ounces of palm kernel oil

4.6 ounces of soybean oil

6.3 ounces of coconut oil

2.3 ounces of cocoa butter

8.4 ounces palm oil

5.1 ounces of sunflower oil

2.7 ounces of castor oil

For the lye solution

6.4 ounces of lye

13 ounces of home brewed fresh green tea

The magic touch

5- 8 tsp of green tea leaves from what you brewed

1.1 ounces of lemongrass essential oil

1.1 ounces of eucalyptus essential oil

COFFEE SOAP RECIPE

One of the most amazing ways to start your morning is with the smell of coffee on your hands. Even if you are running late and couldn't drink your coffee, you can still make it through the day by using this soap recipe. You can use the standard soap recipe; however, you can replace the water in the lye solution with freshly brewed coffee rather than purely water. You can use half the allocated weight of water as coffee or use it entirely as coffee. You can add freshly ground 1-2 teaspoons of coffee for each pound of soap as a powerful exfoliant. Follow the usual cold process soap making steps. Add the ingredients titled under "the magic touch" at trace. Let your wonder soap cure for 3-4 weeks. The peppermint oil compliments the smell of coffee beautifully and sensually.

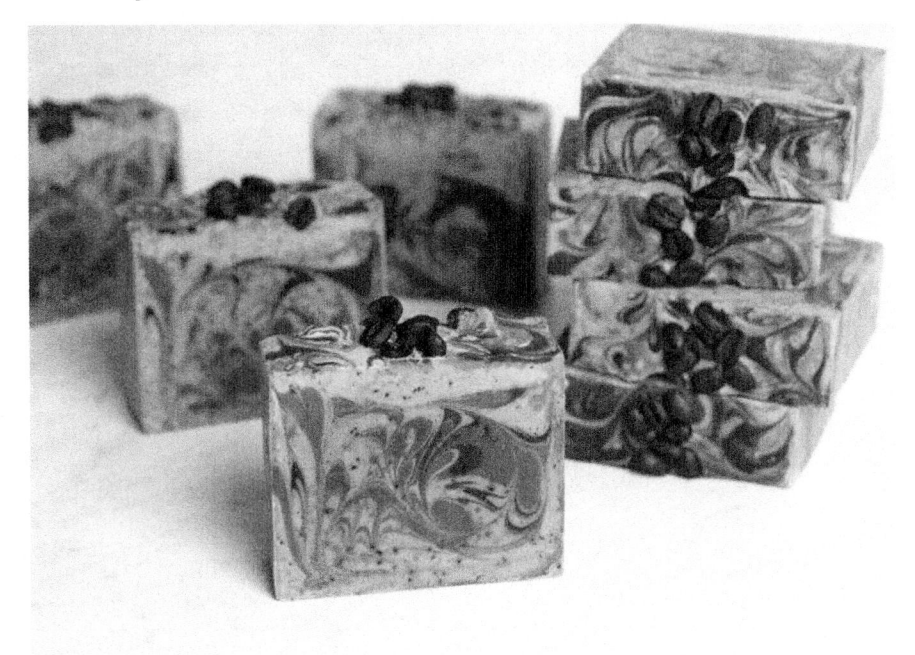

The oils

6.5 ounces of coconut oil

7.5 ounces of olive oil

6.5 ounces of palm oil

1.3 ounces of castor oil

The Lye Mixture

3.1 ounces of lye

8 ounces water (split to 4 oz. of water and 4 coffee or substitute with 8 oz of coffee

The magic touch

1-2 tsp of Ground Coffee

1 ounce of peppermint oil (optional)

Healthy Classical Pine Tar soap

Pine tar is one of the classical ingredients in soap due to its health benefits on the skin such as fighting eczema and other skin conditions. Pine tar has a wood like smell with a gooey appearance. You can create a water bath for a glass dish that contains the pine tar to make it more liquid. Be careful with using this recipe for commercial purposes as you become legally responsible for creating a drug responsible for medical treatment rather than a cosmetic product which requires lots of health regulation and testing to be compliant with consumer protection laws.

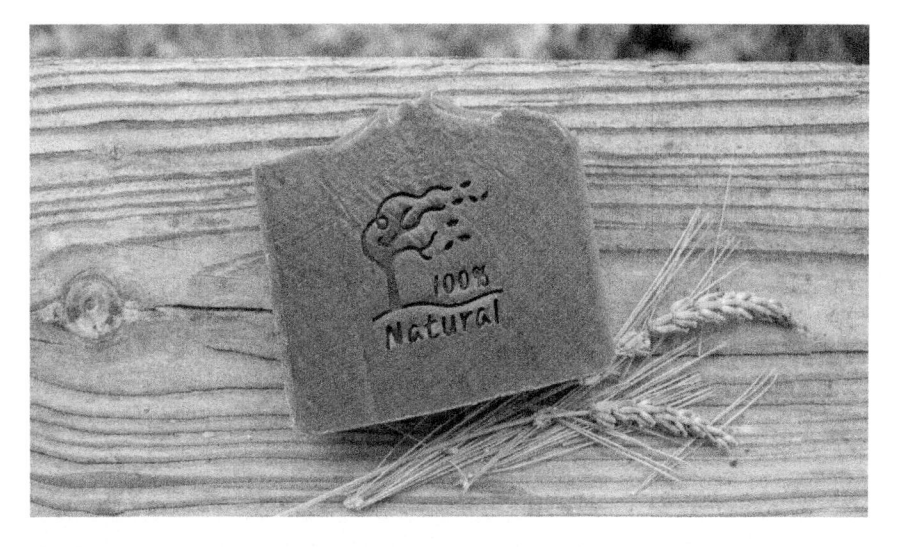

The Oils

8.2 ounces of Palm kernel oil

13.5 ounces of Lard

13.5 ounces of Olive oil

5.8 ounces of Sunflower oil

7.1 ounces of Pine tar (added to the oils)

For the Lye Mixture

5.9 ounces of Lye

15.8 ounces of water (1 tbsp. sugar added to it)

The Magic Touch

Blend 2.5 ounces of Essential oils such as tea tree, lavender, tea tree, eucalyptus

Pampering Shea and Cocoa Butter Recipe

If you wish to nurture your skin with some luxurious soap, you go for the luxurious products that contain nourishing elements such as cocoa butter or shea butter. Why do this when you can do this at home and control everything. This recipe uses double butter for extreme nourishment to your skin.

This recipe makes about 3 pounds of soap

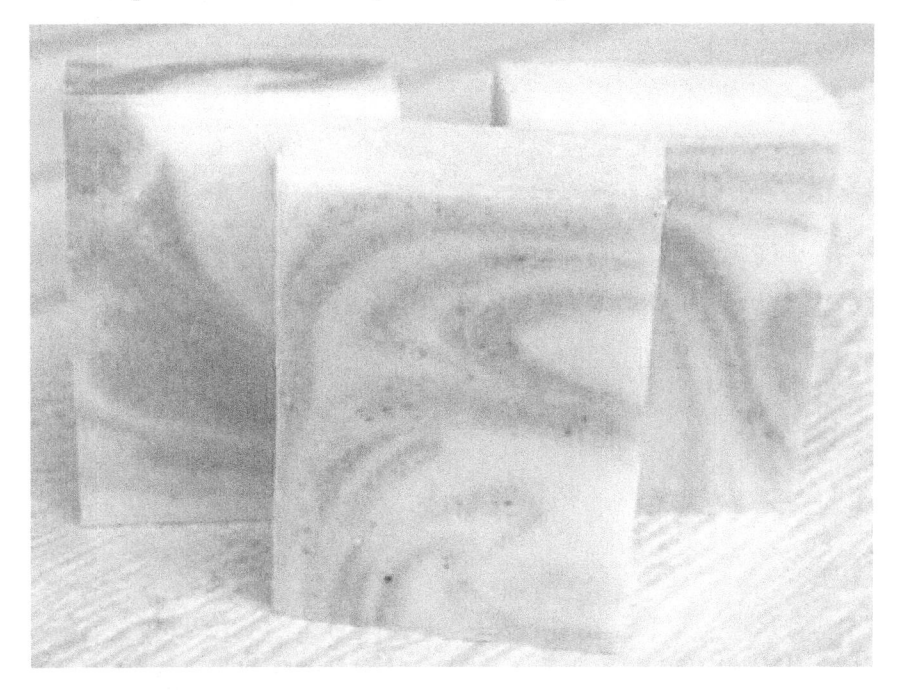

The Oils

5.4 ounces of Shea butter

4.5 ounces of lard

11.2 ounces olive oil

2.2 ounces castor oil

5.8 ounces of cocoa butter

15.6 ounces of coconut oil

For the Lye Solution

6.3 ounces lye

12.6 ounces water

Personal Touch

2 ounces of any fragrance or essential oil blend

Golden or light brown

Pumpkin Spice Soap

Pumpkin style soap for fall.

With the approach of fall, this would be the perfect recipe to delve into. The refreshing smell of pumpkin spice will be an absolute gorgeous addition to your bathroom.

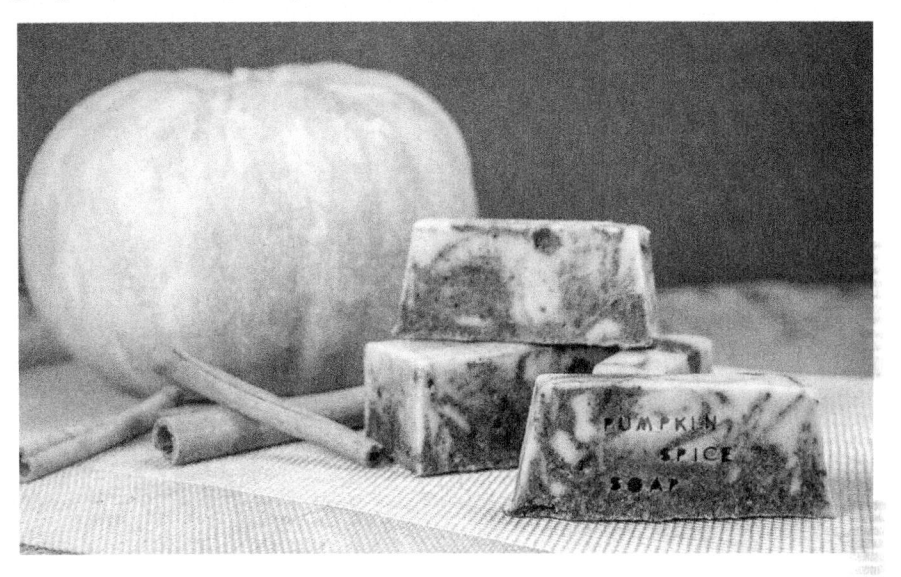

The Oils

12.8 ounces of Coconut Oil

5.1 ounces of Sunflower Oil

15.3 ounces of Olive Oil

15.3 ounces of Lard

2.5 ounces of Castor Oil

For the Lye Solution

7.2 ounces of Lye

15 ounces of water (Add 2 tsp of sugar and 1.5 tsp of salt)

The Magic Touch

3 tsp. of pumpkin pie spice (optional but preferred)

2 ounces of Pumpkin Pie fragrance oil

(Optional) 2 ounces of finely chopped canned pumpkin

Goat Milk with coloured Glitter

One of the most attractive and easy to make soap is goat milk soap, which will be white in colour, perfect in consistency that is designed with sparkling glitter and quartz stones of your choice. You can choose to make this soap sparkling with blue and violet with brown and white glitter to make the universe or you can make a glittery sea with blue dye and golden glitter. It is all your choice with this recipe.

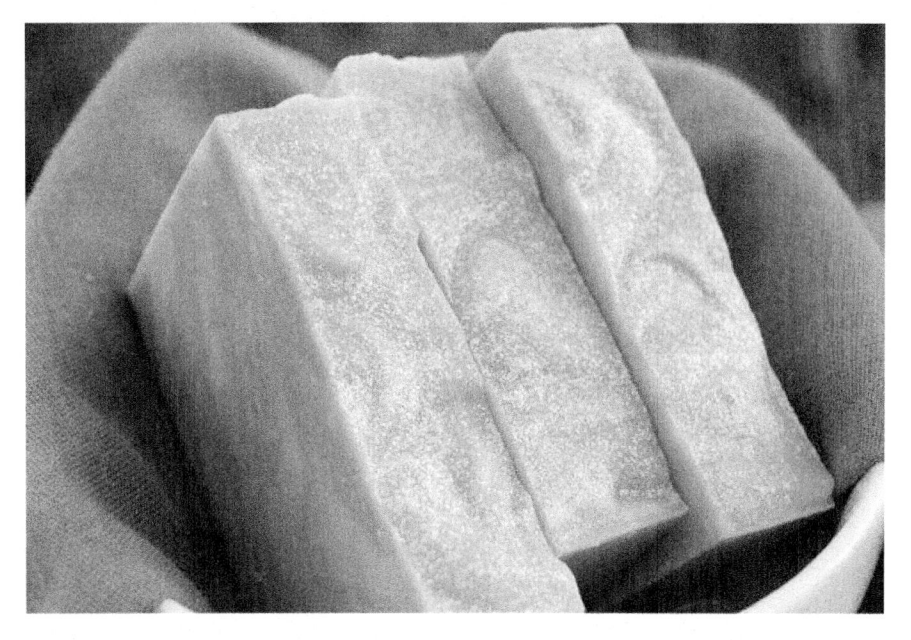

The Oils

1 ounce of castor oil

2.1 ounces of canola oil

5.2 ounces of palm oil

6.3 ounces of coconut oil

6.3 ounces of olive oil

For the Lye Solution

3 ounces of lye

7.2 ounces of goat milk

Additional (Add during trace)

1 table spoon of glitter of your favorite colour

1 tea spoon of orange fragrance oil

1 table spoon of decorative quartz added to the surface of the soap

Refreshing and Soothing Cucumber Blend

Cucumber is known for its natural soothing effects of the skin. Making soap with cucumber instead of water is one of the most wonderful additions and recipes you can try. You can also avoid using a color dye as this soap will have a splendid semi-transparent green color due to the cucumber.

This recipe makes 2 pounds of soap

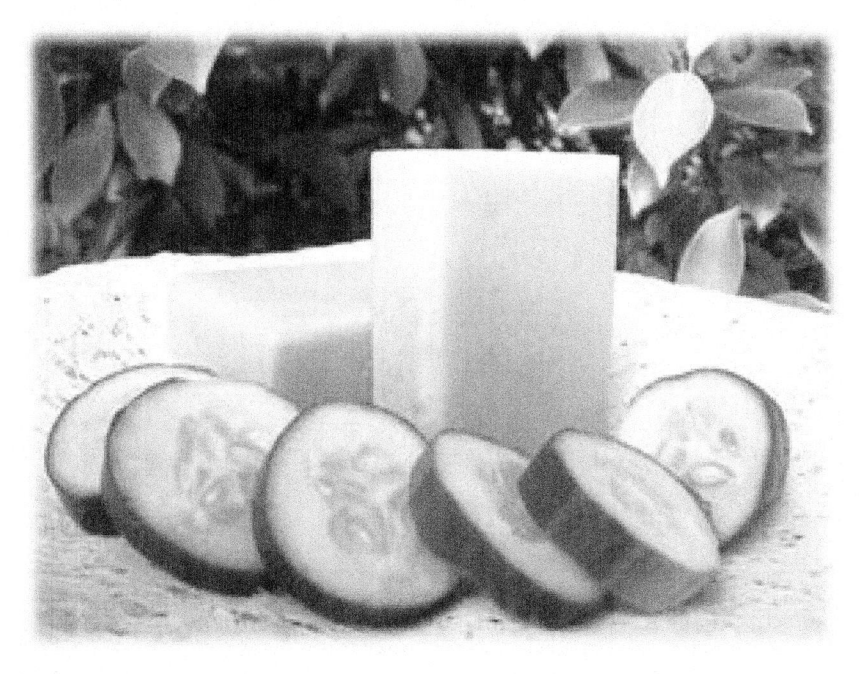

The Oils

7 ounces of Palm Oil

7.5 ounces of Olive Oil

1.5 ounces of Cocoa Butter

7.5 ounces of Coconut Oil

1.5 ounces of Castor Oil

For the Lye Solution

7.5 ounces of completely liquid cucumber, peel of the skin

3.6 ounces of lye

The Magic Touch

To gain green specks in your soap, finely grind/grate cucumber with its peel

The cucumber juice will add a natural colour to this soap recipe

Coconut Milk Soap

One of the wonderful additions you can add to your soap is using coconut milk in your soap. It has moisturizing qualities and increases your skin youth and softness.

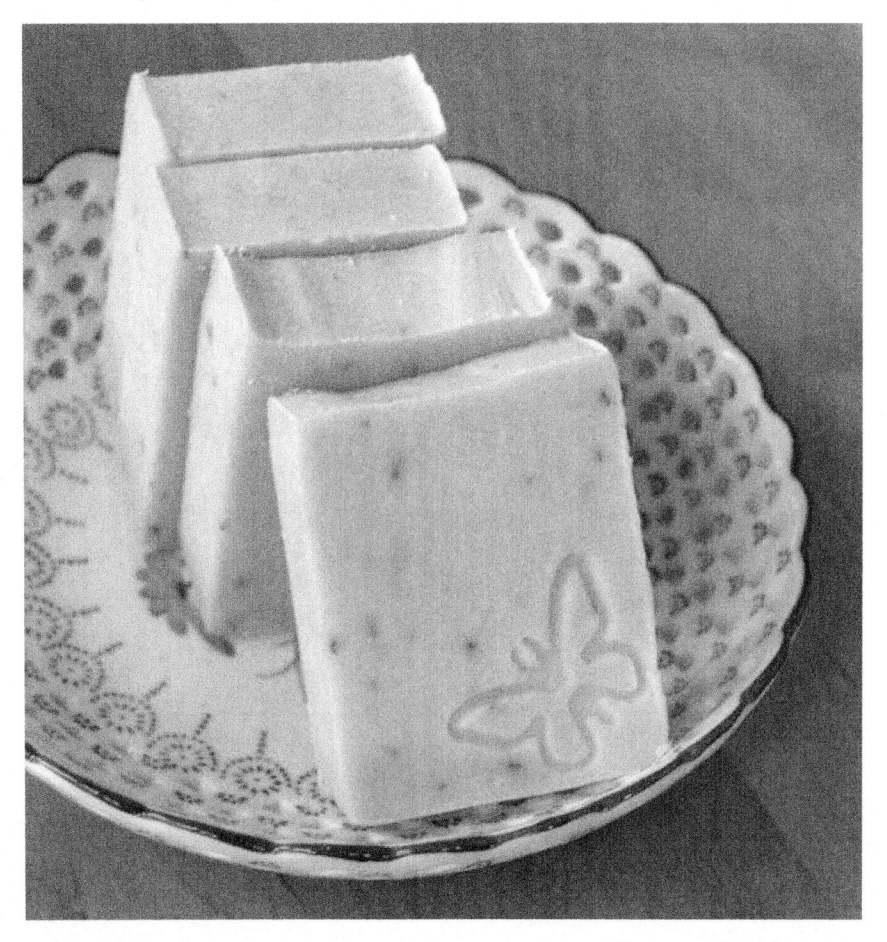

The Oils

1 ounce of castor oil

2.1 ounces of canola oil

5.2 ounces of palm oil

6.3 ounces of coconut oil

6.3 ounces of olive oil

For the Lye Solution

3 ounces of lye

7.2 ounces of coconut milk

Additional

1 ounce of fragrance oil

Tea Tree and Charcoal Soap

The wonderful properties of charcoal makes this soap very healthy to the skin. Charcoal absorbs oil, pulls it out of the pores and binds with it. Think of the cleaning properties of this soap. The tea tree oil blends perfectly with charcoal and is perfect for oily skin.

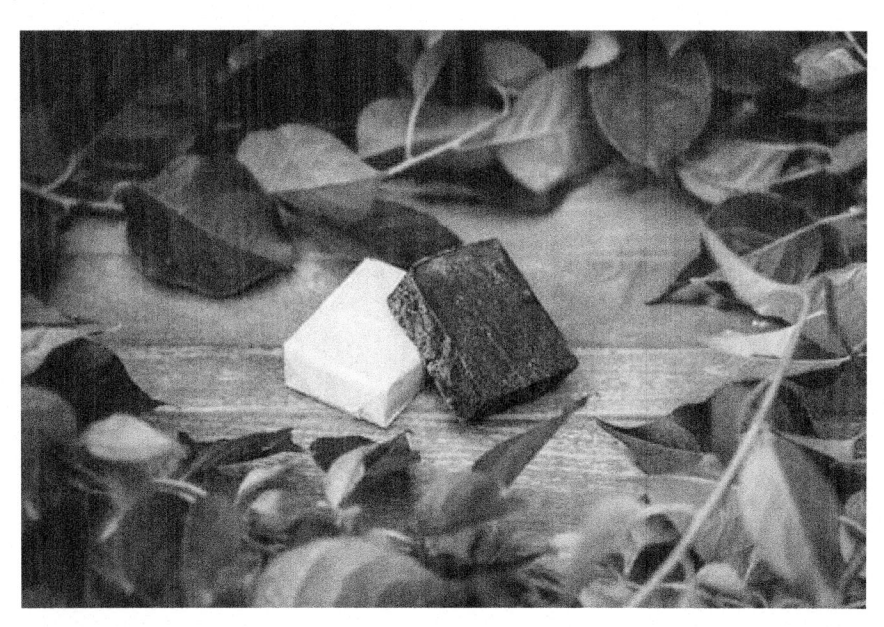

The Oils

14.5 ounces of Olive Oil

9 ounces of Coconut Oil

1.8 ounces of Tamanu Oil

9 ounces of Palm Oil

1.7 ounces of Castor Oil

For the Lye Mixture

5.1 ounces of Sodium Hydroxide Lye

10.1 ounces of Distilled Water (15% water discount)

The Magic Touch (Added during trace)

1.7 ounce of Tea Tree Essential Oil

2 Table spoons of Activated Charcoal

CLOVER AND ALOE

Sometimes it is best to stray from the ordinary and try new and unique recipes. Clover is not a commonly used fragrance in soap, but it is such an underrated one. You can make your soap unique with this perfect oil blend and clover and aloe fragranced soap.

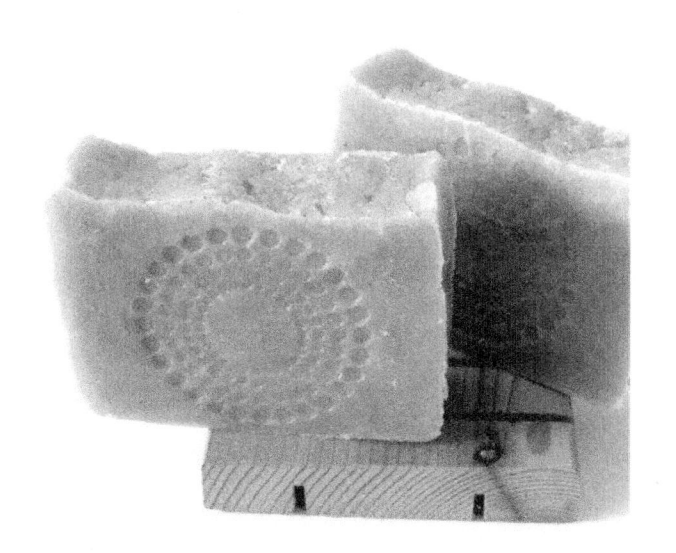

The Oils

3.2 ounces of Sweet Almond Oil

4 ounces of Rice Bran Oil

16 ounces of Canola Oil

0.8 ounces of Castor Oil

8 ounces of Palm Oil

8 ounces of Coconut Oil

For the Lye Mixture

5.5 ounces of Lye

13.2 ounces of Water

The Magic Touch (Added during trace)

2.3 ounces of Clover and Aloe Fragrance Oil

Colorant of your choice

Coconut Oil Soap (Beginners recipe)

This soap gives a lot of lather which is very satisfying. If you are a beginner, this soap is quite easy and enticing to try as it only makes use of oil, making it simple and quick.

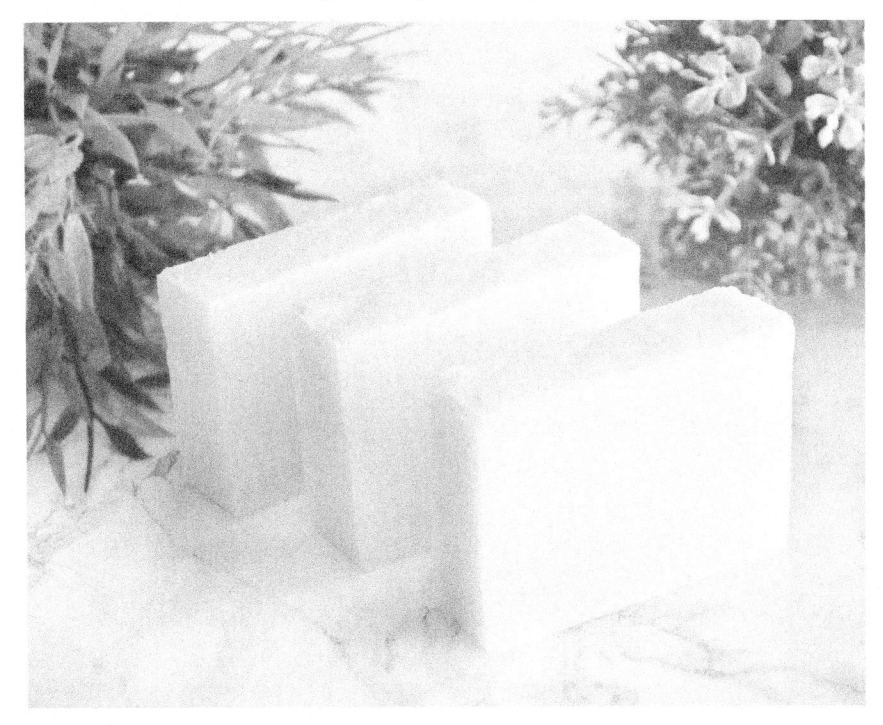

The Oil (Single oil recipe)

33 ounces coconut oil

For the Lye Mixture

4.83 ounces of lye

12.54 oz water

Additional

1.3 ounce of your favorite essential oils

Lavender and Goat Milk Soap

Goat Milk soap is one of my favorite soaps to use due to its perfect consistency and wonderful white color that allows you to contrast anything with it, such as lavender leaves or purple swirls in this recipe.

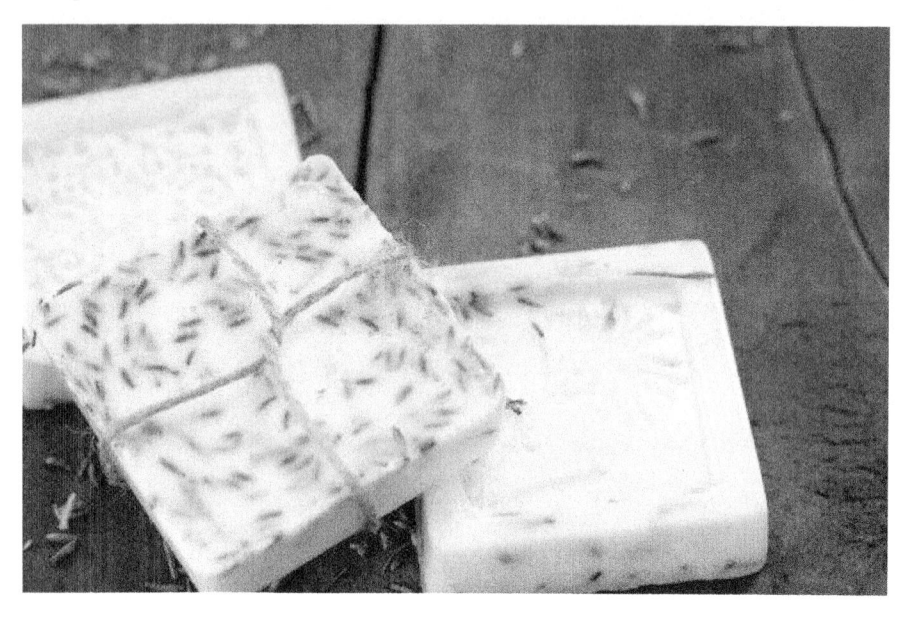

The Oils

1 ounce of castor oil

2.1 ounces of canola oil

5.2 ounces of palm oil

6.3 ounces of coconut oil

6.3 ounces of olive oil

For the Lye Solution

3 ounces of lye

7.2 ounces of goat milk

Additional

0.5 teaspoon of lavender fragrance oil

1 tablespoon of dried lavender flowers

OAT MEAL SOAP

Oats are a skin friendly natural grain, perfect for exfoliating as well whitening. Oat meal in your soap is such a wonderful and luxurious touch to add to your soap.

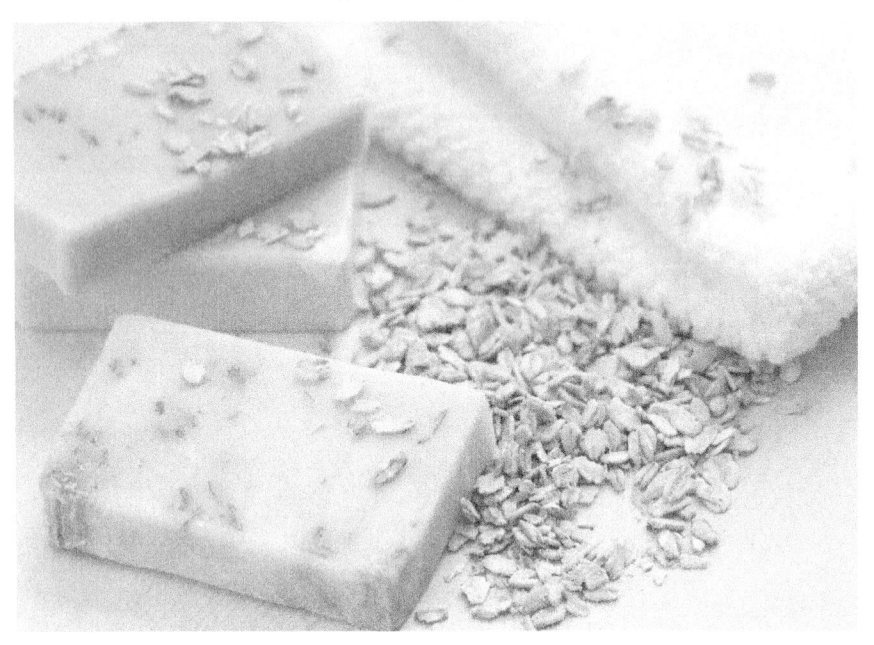

The oils

2.75 ounces 14% almond oil

1 ounce 5% castor oil

5.3 ounces 27% olive oil

5.3 ounces 27% palm oil

5.3 ounces 27% coconut oil

For the Lye solution

2.8 ounces of lye

5.9 ounces of goat milk

The Magic Touch

1 ounce lavender fragrance oil

3-4 tablespoons of oats

(optional) Dried lavender flowers

ZESTY LEMON SOAP

Some people go crazy for the smell of fresh lemon. If you are one of those people, you will enjoy this lemon fragranced soap. Moreover, the lemon zests in this recipe will add a cute touch to your soap.

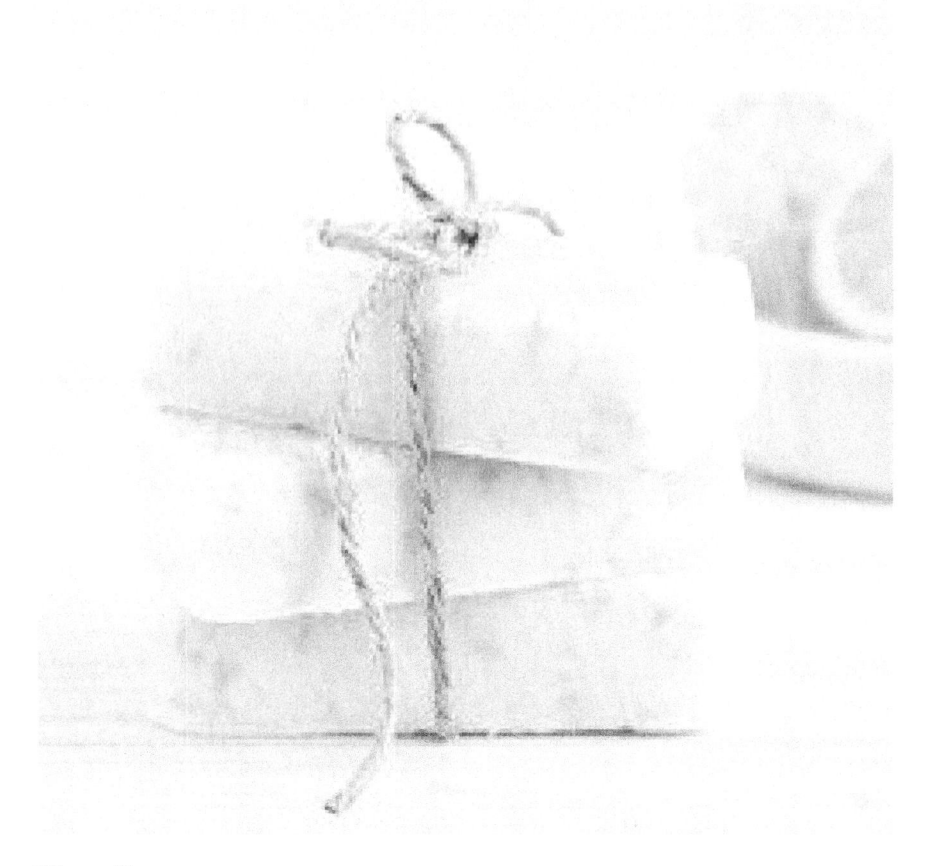

The oils

7.5 ounces olive oil

6.5 ounces palm oil

1.3 ounces castor oil

6.5 ounces coconut oil

The Lye Mixture

3.1 ounces lye

8 ounces water

The Magic Touch

1 ounce of lemon fragrance oil or essential oil

1 tablespoon of grated lemon zest (mix with the soap at trace or spray on top or both)

ORANGE ZEST SOAP

Some people go crazy for the smell of fresh orange. If you are one of those people, you will enjoy this orange fragranced soap. Moreover, the orange zests in this recipe will add a cute touch to your soap.

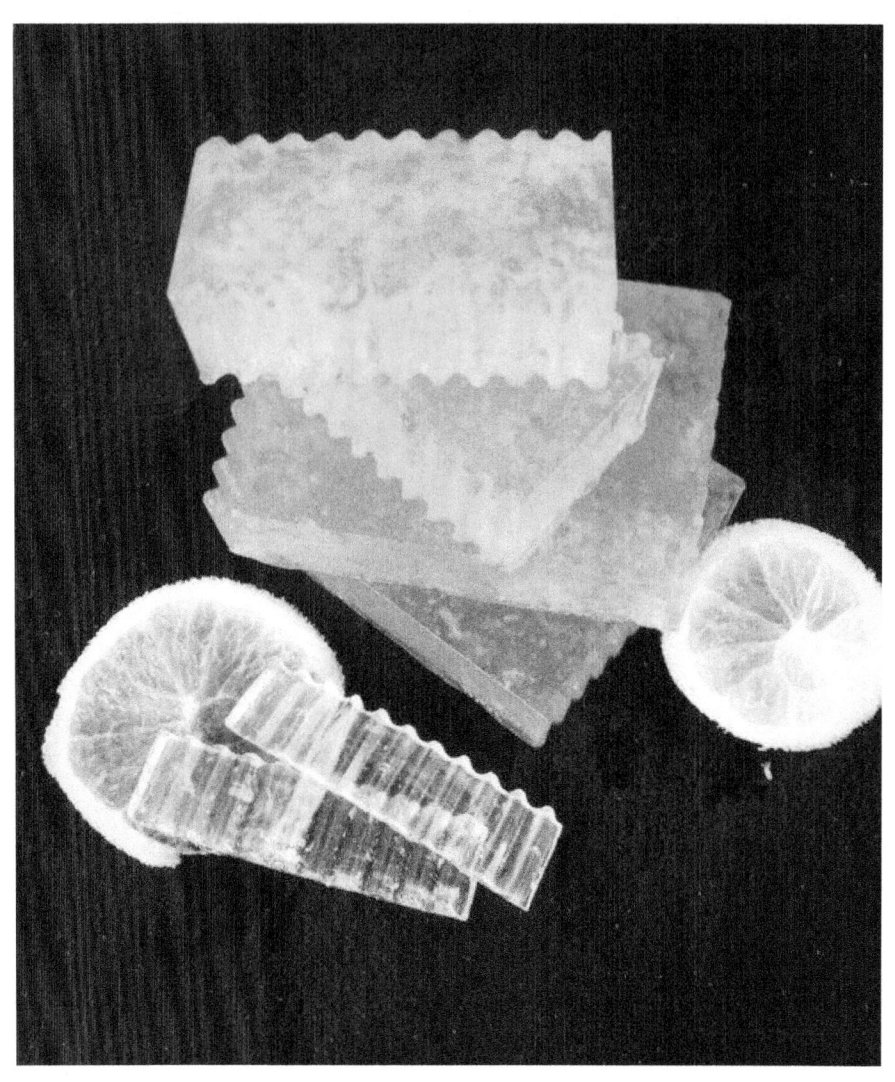

The Oils

7 ounces of Palm Oil

7.5 ounces of Olive Oil

1.5 ounces of Cocoa Butter

7.5 ounces of Coconut Oil

1.5 ounces of Castor Oil

For the Lye Solution

7.5 ounces of water

3.6 ounces of lye

The Magic Touch

1 ounce Orange fragrance or essential oil

1-2 table spoons of orange zest

TEA AND PEPPERMINT SOAP

If tea with peppermint is one of your favorite things to have in the morning or at night, you can extend your joy by making tea and peppermint soap so that you can enjoy the smell in the morning and at night.

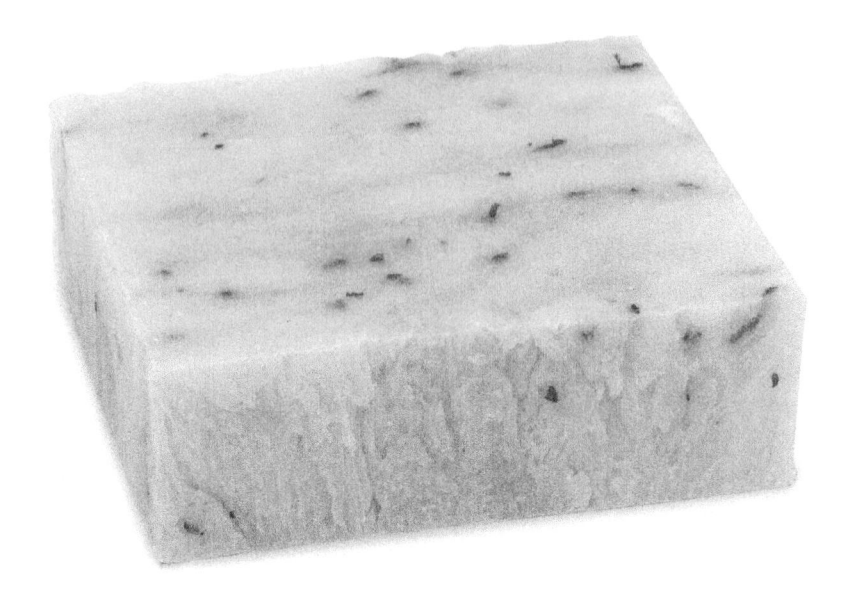

The oils

11 ounces of olive oil

5.2 ounces of palm kernel oil

4.6 ounces of soybean oil

6.3 ounces of coconut oil

2.3 ounces of cocoa butter

8.4 ounces palm oil

5.1 ounces of sunflower oil

2.7 ounces of castor oil

For the lye solution

6.4 ounces of lye

13 ounces of home brewed fresh tea

The magic touch

6 tsp of tea leaves from what you brewed

1.1 ounces of peppermint essential oil

FRENCH GREEN CLAY SOAP

Taking your soap to the next level would mean including new ingredients. French clay is perfect for the skin, adding it to your soap is such a luxurious touch and takes your soap making skills to the next level.

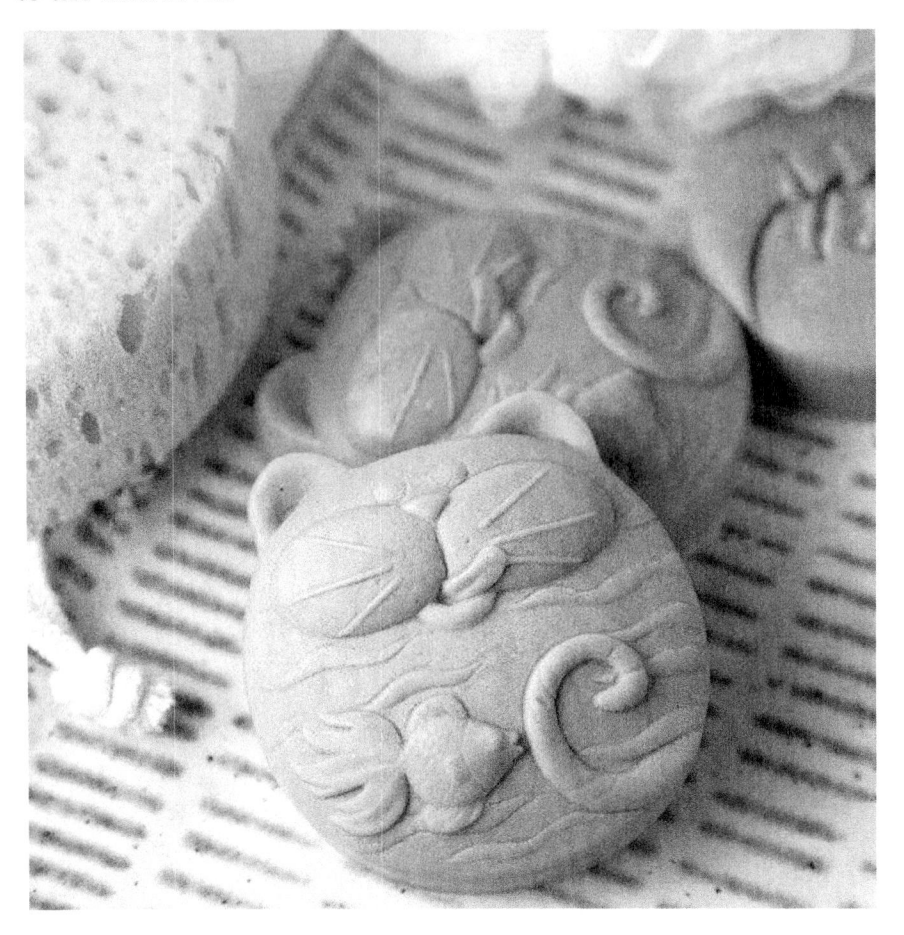

The Oils

1 ounce of castor oil

2.1 ounces of canola oil

5.2 ounces of palm oil

6.3 ounces of coconut oil

6.3 ounces of olive oil

For the Lye Solution

3 ounces of lye

7.2 ounces of goat's milk

The Magic Touch

1 ounce of any earthy fragrance oil

4-8 tablespoons of French green clay (you can add more based on how much clay you want in your soap)

Vanilla Soap

Vanilla fans out there would agree that vanilla fragranced soap is a wonderful addition to their bathroom or merch. You can't be making soap without having tried the vanilla fragranced soap.

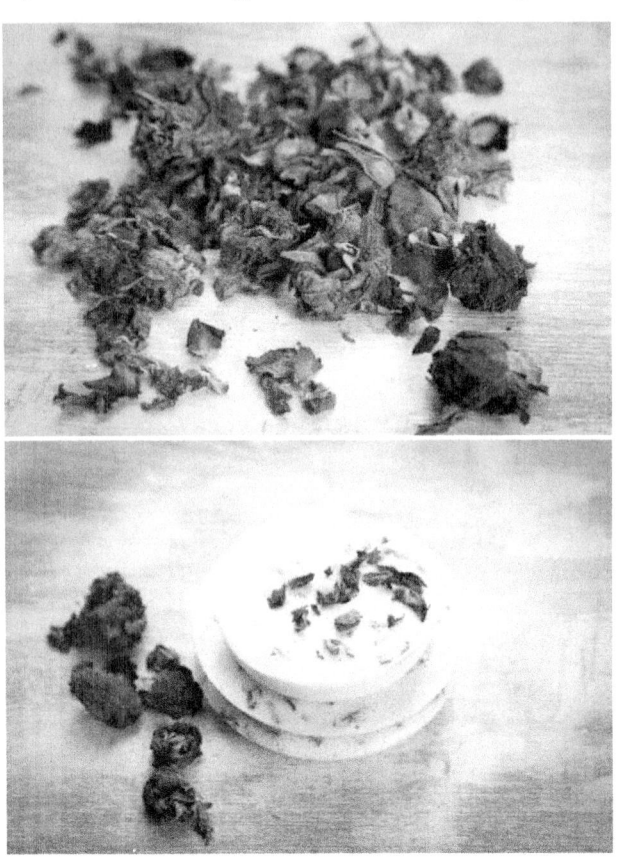

The oils

7.5 ounces olive oil

6.5 ounces palm oil

1.3 ounces castor oil

6.5 ounces coconut oil

The Lye Mixture

3.1 ounces lye

8 ounces water

Personal Additions

1 ounce of Vanilla fragrance oil or essential oil blend

A handful of Rose Petals

ROSE WATER PETAL SOAP

Rose water is one of the best things you can put on your skin. It softens and tones the skin. It would be wonderful if you make your soap with rose water instead of regular water. You can add rose petals for luxury.

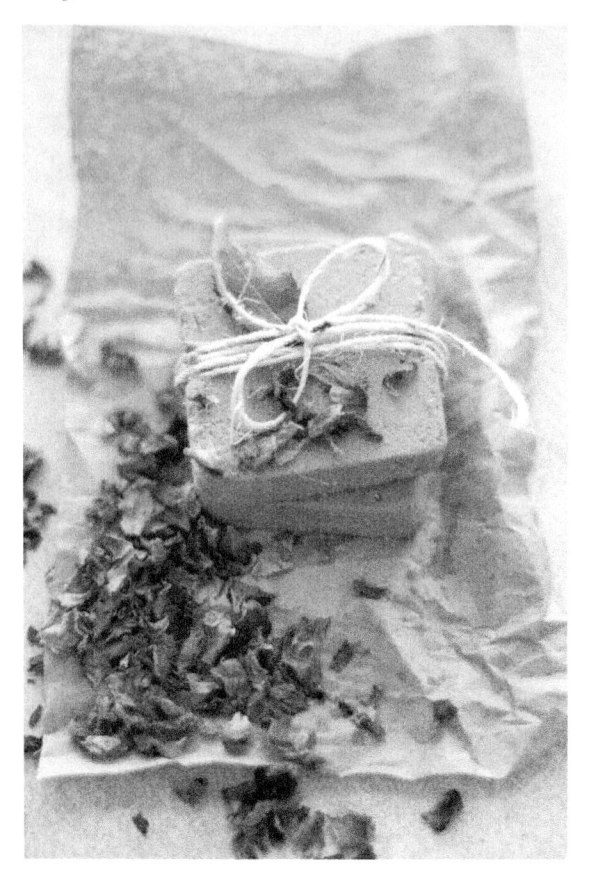

The Oils

6.5 ounces of coconut oil

7.5 ounces of olive oil

6.5 ounces of palm oil

1.3 ounces of castor oil

The Lye Mixture

3.1 ounces of lye

8 ounces Rose water

The Magic Touch

1 tsp of Rose essential oil

Red rose petals (as desired)

Sea Mud and Cedar Wood Soap

There is a perfect persona and mood for this soap. It has all the skin benefits of sea mud while being fragranced like cedar wood, a combination that unites you with Mother Nature.

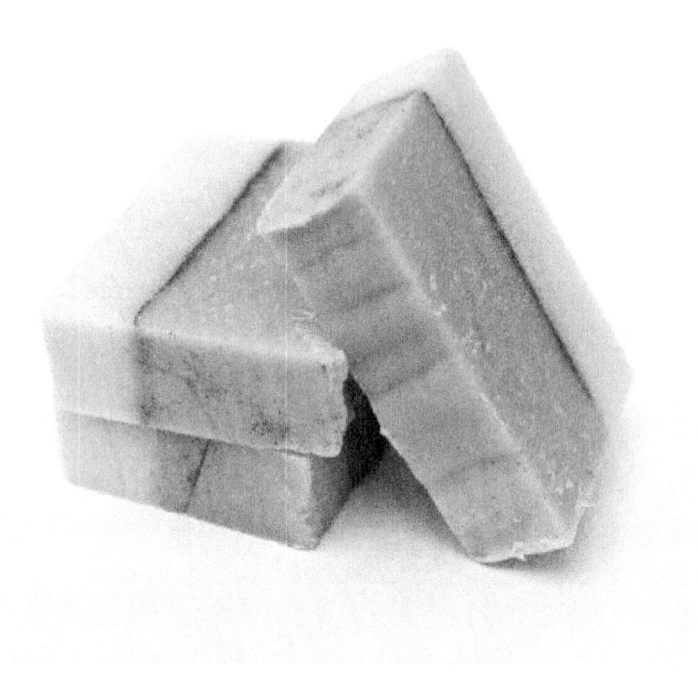

The Oils

20 ounces of olive oil

10 ounces coconut oil

The Lye Mixture

11.4 ounce of water

4.2 ounce of lye

The Magic Touch

2 tablespoons of Sea Mud

1 teaspoon of Cedarwood essential oil

1 teaspoon Rosemary essential oil

CHAI VANILLA SOAP

You can always get creative with your additions to soap. In this recipe, we make use of the goat milk so that you get a white canvas to paint on. In this recipe we will use chai tea leaves to decorate the soap and vanilla fragrance to complement it.

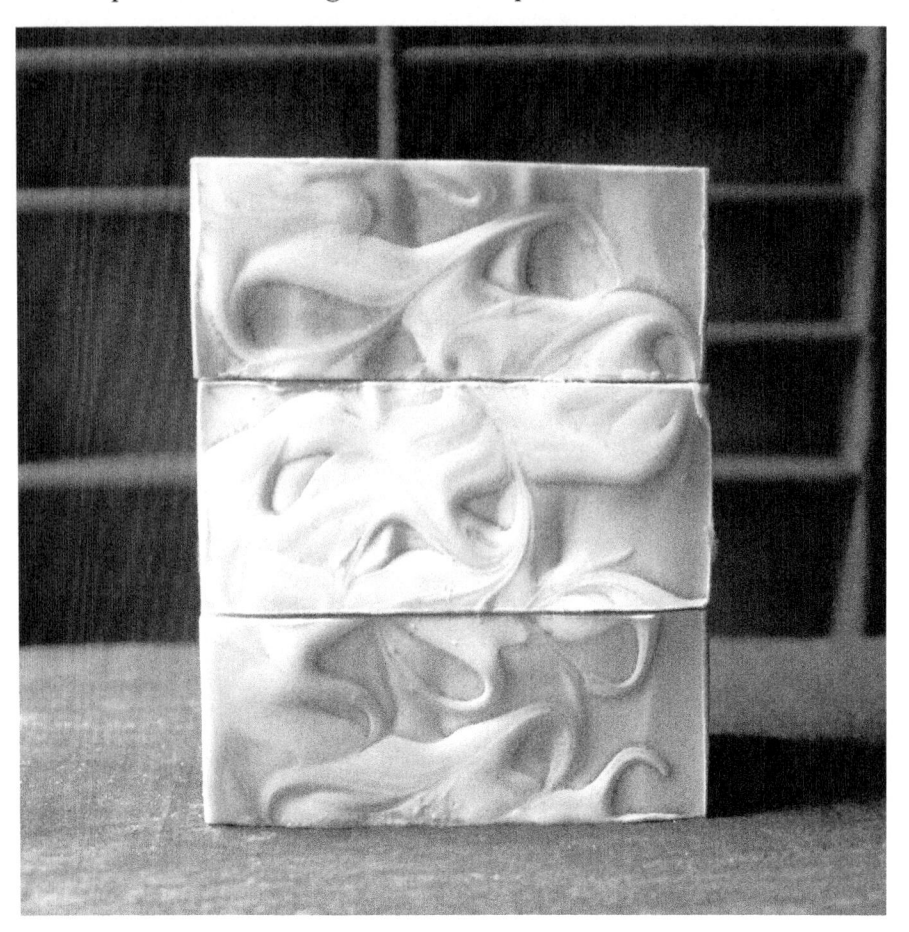

The Oils

1 ounce of castor oil

2.1 ounces of canola oil

5.2 ounces of palm oil

6.3 ounces of coconut oil

6.3 ounces of olive oil

For the Lye Solution

3 ounces of lye

7.2 ounces of goat's milk

Additional

Few bags or 2-4 table spoons of Chai Tea

1 teaspoon of vanilla essential oil

APPLE CINNAMON WINTER SOAP

This is one of my favorite soaps because it combines apple and cinnamon, such a wonderful combination. The warm mix of apple and cinnamon reminds me of the warm apple pie in winter that is why I call this a winter recipe. You can always fragrance your soap with these two ingredients or add pieces of apples and cinnamon powder as well.

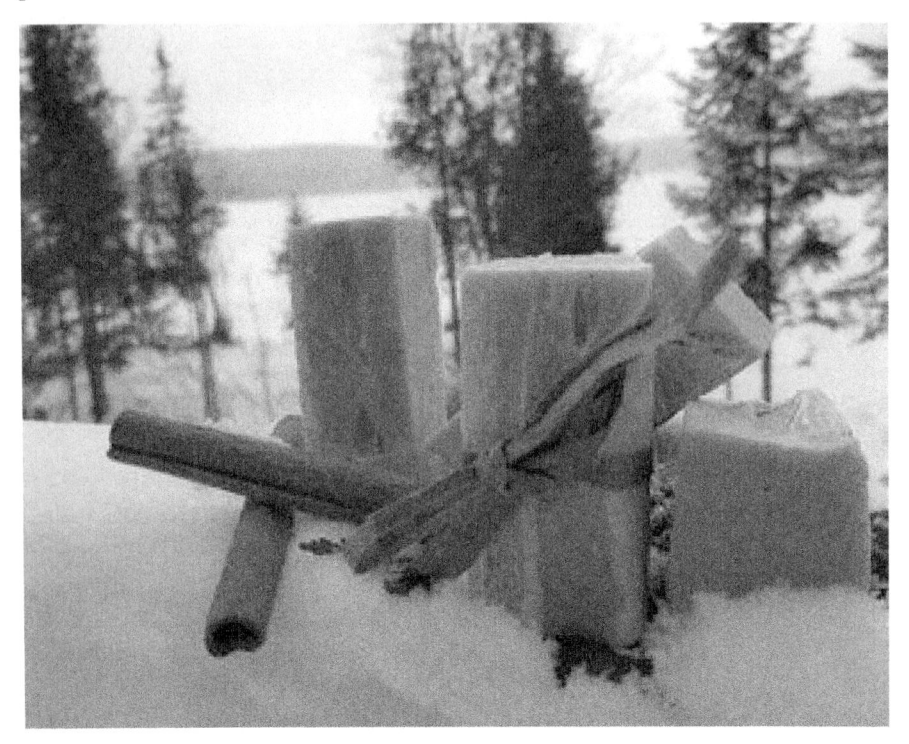

The Oils

1 ounce of castor oil

2.1 ounces of canola oil

5.2 ounces of palm oil

6.3 ounces of coconut oil

6.3 ounces of olive oil

For the Lye Solution

3 ounces of lye

7.2 ounces of goat's milk

Additional

1 tablespoon of freshly and finely ground cinnamon

1 teaspoon of apple fragrance/essential oil

LOOFA SOAP

How convenient would it be if your soap was molded on your bath sponge immediately, so you can just wet it and use it right away. This recipe offers you a creative and distinctive way to represent and use your soap.

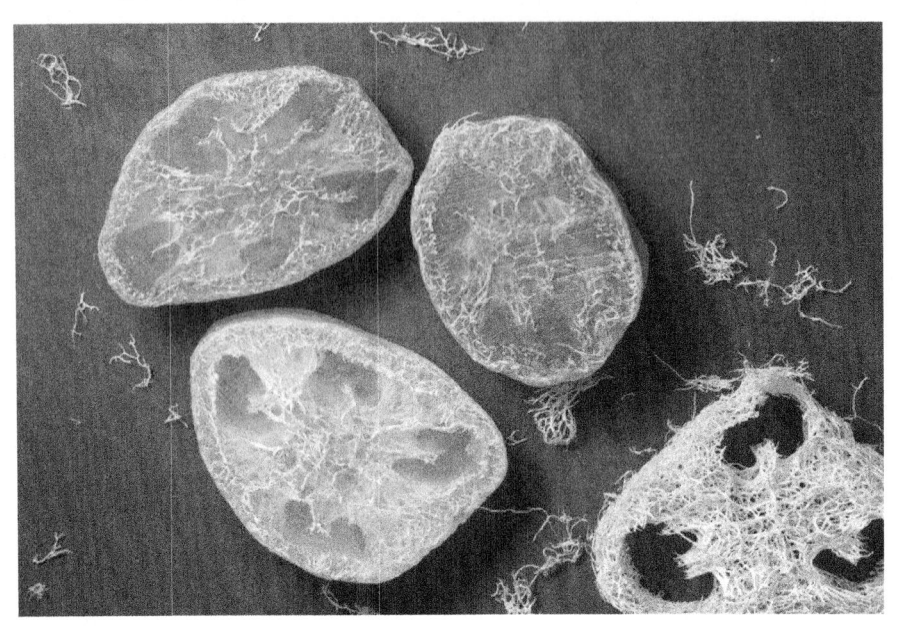

The oils

7.5 ounces olive oil

6.5 ounces palm oil

1.3 ounces castor oil

6.5 ounces coconut oil

The Lye Mixture

3.1 ounces lye

8 ounces water

Personal Additions

1 ounces of your favorite essential oil blend

A beautiful soap colorant of your choice

A long loofa (A classic style of sponges, can be found online)

Note: The loofa replaces the mold, you slice the loofa into thin slices and pour the soap on it to create small slices of loofa soap.

Yogurt and Banana Flax Seed Soap

Yogurt and banana are amongst some of the most moisturizing ingredients you can use on your skin. This recipe combines the yogurt and banana with flax seeds in a unique and healthy blend that is perfect for your skin. S

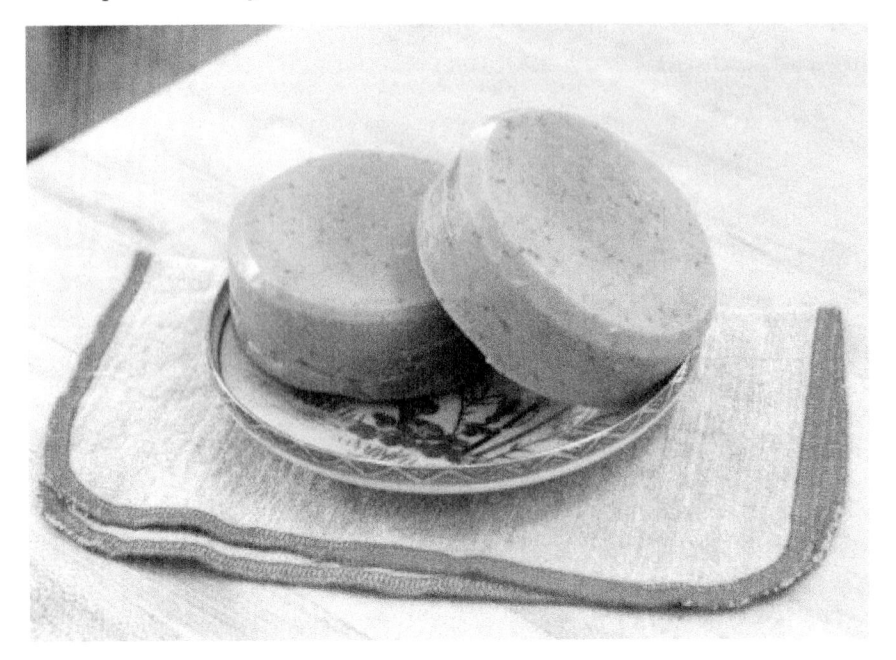

The Oils

17.6 ounces of olive oil

1.6 ounces of castor oil

4.8 ounces of babassu oil

3.2 ounces of cocoa butter

1.6 ounces of organic flax seed oil

1.6 ounces of coconut oil

1.6 ouncse of Shea butter

The Lye Mixture

4.25 ounces of lye

9.75 ounces of water

Magic Additions

1 teaspoon of yogurt powder (added to the oil)

1.5 teaspoon of banana powder (added to the oil)

2 ounces of your favorite fragrance oil

LEMON AND POPPY SOAP

Another creative blend is this lemon fragranced soap that is decorated with poppy seeds. The lemon has antibacterial properties that makes your soap pretty and useful.

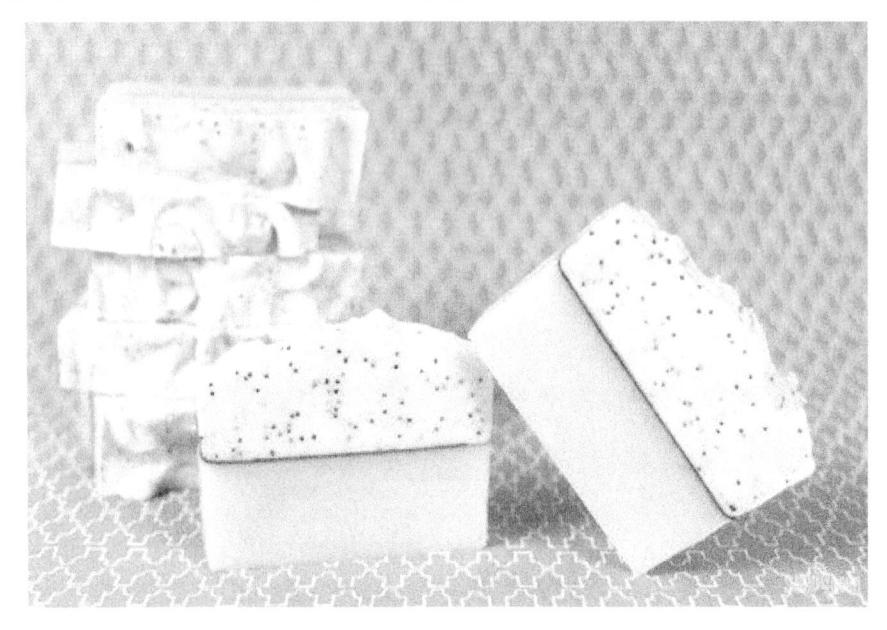

The Oils

1 ounce of castor oil

2.1 ounces of canola oil

5.2 ounces of palm oil

6.3 ounces of coconut oil

6.3 ounces of olive oil

For the Lye Solution

3 ounces of lye

7.2 ounces of goat's milk

The Magic Touch

1 teaspoon of lemon fragrance

2 tablespoons of lemon zest

1 tablespoon of poppy seeds

Raspberry Soap

One of my favorite additions and recipes is raspberry soap. The aroma and color of raspberries is a wonderful addition to any soap. Raspberry also has antioxidant properties, that is why, you can add it to your soap for its benefit.

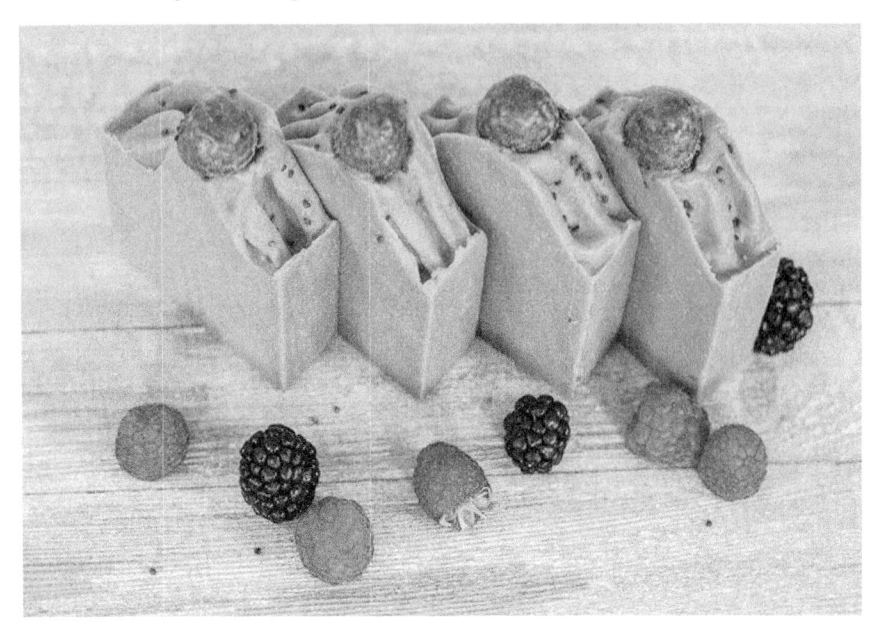

The Oils

1 ounce of castor oil

2.1 ounces of canola oil

5.2 ounces of palm oil

6.3 ounces of coconut oil

6.3 ounces of olive oil

For the Lye Solution

3 ounces of lye

7.2 ounces of goat's milk

The Magic Touch

1 teaspoon of raspberry fragrance

2 ounces of freshly diced raspberries

Conclusion

It is a great experience to try new things. If you haven't tried Do It Yourself homemade soap, it is best that you try this interesting hobby now. We hope this book has been your handy guide in shedding light on the different corners of homemade soap and guided you on how to start, how to proceed and how to create visually appealing and beautifully smelling bars of soap that exfoliate or nourish your skin. Moreover, we have used a handful of recipes so that you can start right away with recipes from a trusted source. Don't be afraid to get creative with new ingredients, color patterns, design and decorations. Soap making is just like cooking. The possibilities are endless. Set your creativity free to explore.

Printed in Great Britain
by Amazon